Hope Donahue grew up in Los Angeles, California, and holds a master's degree in journalism from the University of California at Berkeley. She was a finalist in *Glimmer Train*'s short story competition, and her short fiction has also appeared in *Other Voices*. She now lives in New Jersey with her husband and their four children.

BEAUTIFUL STRANGER

A Memoir of an Obsession with Perfection

HOPE DONAHUE

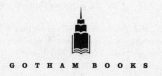

GOTHAM BOOKS

GOTHAM BOOKS
Published by Penguin Group (USA) Inc.
375 Hudson Street, New York, New York 10014, U.S.A.
Penguin Group (Canada), 10 Alcorn Avenue, Toronto, Ontario, Canada M4V 3B2
(a division of Pearson Penguin Canada Inc.); Penguin Books Ltd, 80 Strand, London
WC2R 0RL, England; Penguin Ireland, 25 St Stephen's Green, Dublin 2, Ireland
(a division of Penguin Books Ltd); Penguin Group (Australia), 250 Camberwell Road,
Camberwell, Victoria 3124, Australia (a division of Pearson Australia Group Pty Ltd);
Penguin Books India Pvt Ltd, 11 Community Centre, Panchsheel Park, New Delhi - 110
017, India; Penguin Group (NZ), cnr Airborne and Rosedale Roads, Albany, Auckland 1310,
New Zealand (a division of Pearson New Zealand Ltd); Penguin Books (South Africa)
(Pty) Ltd, 24 Sturdee Avenue, Rosebank, Johannesburg 2196, South Africa

Penguin Books Ltd, Registered Offices: 80 Strand, London WC2R 0RL, England

Published by Gotham Books, a division of Penguin Group (USA) Inc.
Previously published as a Gotham Books hardcover edition.

First Gotham trade paperback printing, August 2005

1   3   5   7   9   10   8   6   4   2

Gotham Books and the skyscraper logo are trademarks of
Penguin Group (USA) Inc.

The Library of Congress has cataloged the hardcover edition of this title as follows:
Donahue, Hope, 1968–
Beautiful stranger : a memoir of an obsession with perfection / by Hope Donahue.
p. cm.
ISBN 1-592-40074-4 (hardcover)   ISBN 1-592-40152-X (paperback)
1. Donahue, Hope, 1968—Mental health. 2. Surgery, Plastic—Patients—
California—Los Angeles—Biography. 3. Compulsive behavior—Patients—
California—Los Angeles—Biography. 4. Surgery, Plastic—Psychological aspects.
5. Beauty, Personal—Psychological aspects. I. Title.
RD118.5.D665   2004
617.9'52'092—dc22   2004004177

Printed in the United States of America
Set in Garamond   Designed by Mia Risberg

For Ray

BEAUTIFUL STRANGER

H ere is what you need to know.

My name is Hope. I am thirty-six years old. I grew up in a tiny enclave of Los Angeles called Hancock Park, an area as renowned for its stately mansions and old-money families as for the La Brea tar pits, which regularly expel relics of bone and tooth from the animals long ago trapped there, lured by a mirage of water.

I am an only child. My father is a bank chairman, my grandfather a doctor of international acclaim. My mother stayed home in our beautiful house to raise me, as mothers did then. I am intelligent, witty, well traveled. I went to the best private schools. I never had to apply for a college scholarship or save for a new car. These things were given to me. I was a debutante. I am five-feet-eight-inches tall, with a model's build, blonde hair, and green eyes. People say I am beautiful.

These are just a few details of my life, but perhaps they are enough to trigger something. Do not be sick with envy at this awe-inspiring list of good fortune. Maybe you've known me, or someone like me. Maybe I was the girl you wanted not to like, because she had so much. The girl whose sunny cheerfulness seemed, you thought, superficial.

Do you remember me now, the girl who had it all?

Dr. S—'s receptionist moves with an aloof, feline grace down the hall. I follow in her wake of Opium, feeling clumsy and inferior, chiding myself at how little it takes to make me feel ungainly and imperfect. At the examining room door she turns to gesture me inside, and I find it hard not to stare at her breasts, which are so high and full they appear to swagger beneath the thin fabric of her top. I want to ask her whether Dr. S— is responsible for them. But it is inappropriate to stare at another woman's breasts, even in the office of a Beverly Hills plastic surgeon renowned for the breasts he creates, so instead I look at the diamond-studded upside-down horseshoe pendant dangling on a chain around her neck. Doesn't she know that wearing the horseshoe this way means that all the good luck is running out?

Alone in the small room, I slip the paper smock over my clothes and struggle to fit my long hair into the paper cap. With the door closed, the silence of the room is so complete and engulfing, I can hear the blood pounding in my ears. The rustle of the paper smock is a roar. The white walls seem to be closing in on me. I want desperately to poke my head out the door, gulp a few breaths of fresh air to divert the flood of panic threatening to overtake me, but I fear looking impatient. Instead I shift uncomfortably on the narrow exam table, feeling the spread of wetness beneath my arms.

Outside the door, a familiar deep male voice rumbles incoherently. My heart gives a lurch of anticipation. Everything changes, now, at the prospect of having Dr. S— so close. Am I his next patient? If not, how much longer will he be? Five minutes? Fifteen? The clock above the door has a mechanical arm that scoots in jerks around its perimeter. Trying to take deep, even breaths, I watch its motion.

Everything in this room is white. I can't help thinking that this feels like a movie in which the recently deceased heroine waits eagerly to meet God, to be judged by Him. Like any good zealot, I expect to be reborn. And then, miraculously, the door clicks open and he enters the room, a tall, good-looking man of about forty-five, as handsome a deity as any Hollywood casting director could have dreamed up, wearing green surgical scrubs which are somewhat rumpled and specked ever so slightly with traces of rusty blood.

"Hope! My dear, good morning. How are you today?"

"Fine," I say, which now that he's here is less of a lie.

Dr. S— approaches me, standing so close I can smell the piney cologne rising off his warm skin. His brows knit together as he studies the bump on my lower lip, a flaw which I know is jarringly obvious in spite of my careful application of matte, flesh-toned lipstick. *Silly,* I think now, *to have applied lipstick; it will be wiped away before Dr. S— can begin his work.*

"We're going to fix this today." He presses the bump and I wince, not only because it hurts, but because I need to see the tender regret in his eyes at having caused me pain. "Sorry. I've got to check a post-op patient, and then we'll begin. It will only be a few more minutes."

When the door closes behind him, I feel I'll jump out of my skin. For the first time, the reality of the procedure hits me: It will hurt, what he's going to do; it's sure to; how could it not hurt? As if the painful bump and my pounding fear are not punishment enough, the familiar blaming refrain descends upon me like a hammer: *This is all your fault. You brought this on yourself. It is your punishment, for wanting something so frivolous, so silly and wasteful. You vain, selfish fool.*

When the door clicks open again, my heart gives a bleat of joy. But it is only the nurse, come to lead me to the operating room.

"Ready?"

She is efficient, perhaps irritated, standing there in her green scrubs. Her plastic name tag, slightly askew, says JEANNE. I follow her down the hallway wishing, childishly and impractically, that she would be kind, perhaps hold my hand. I need some maternal kindness to calm the whoosh of fear in me.

"Hope." Dr. S— steps through the door of his surgical suite, blocking my view of the brightly lit room. "Before we begin, there's something I want to show you. Come in."

To my surprise, there is a woman on the operating table. She is dark-haired, doe-eyed, perhaps forty. Her body is draped in a white blanket. She blinks at me and smiles sleepily.

"Hello," I offer, not knowing what else to say.

"This is Alix," Dr. S— says.

On either side of the white paper sheet beneath her head are a half-dozen or so nickel-sized reddish blotches, where blood from an unseen wound has dripped and been absorbed, then dried.

"Alix just had what I like to call a 'lunchtime lift.' Have you heard of it?"

"No."

"It's revolutionary," he says. "State-of-the-art. It gives the effect of a brow lift without any of the downtime." There's a surge of bravado in Dr. S—'s voice, the voice of a showman, a salesman? I have no interest in a brow lift, so I do not know how to react. Dr. S— approaches the woman on the table, pressing one of her manicured hands in his own. "Come closer, Hope," he scolds gently. "Don't be so shy."

"Sorry." I chuckle nervously. The hushed, private atmosphere of the operating room feels like entering a church, or a stranger's bedroom. And I feel a tinge of annoyance, too: *This is supposed to be my surgery, my moment.* But at Dr. S—'s bidding, I come and stand beside Alix. She turns toward Dr. S—, to whom she gives a languorous look; a look which suggests, in effect with the damp hair at her temples, that she has just awoken not from surgery but from a short sleep after having made love. Dr. S— gently lifts the hair above her right temple, revealing a startling line of black stitches against the white skin of her scalp. She winces, and he quickly smoothes her hair back into place, then strokes the dewy skin of her forehead, once, with the back of his fingers. She smiles up at him, and the look of trust and intimacy they exchange makes my throat ache with longing.

"Just *look* at her," Dr. S— says to me, his eyes still fixed on Alix. "Isn't she lovely? She looks twenty-five years old."

My smile, automatic, hides my confusion. I myself am only twenty-three years old.

"You could benefit from this too, Hope." Dr. S— replaces Alix's hand on her blue-smocked chest, then turns the full wattage of his gaze on me. His body radiates a warmth in the cool, sterile operating room. "You're very girl-next-door, and this would give you an exotic, sort of foreign look. Here, let me show you."

Exotic. Foreign. He may not have sold me on the prospect of a brow lift, but these are promises that entice. How can I resist a delicious, illicit offer to become someone I am not? Does Dr. S— see inside me, does he know that if I could, I would shed my face and body, my very self, on his table as nimbly as a snake sheds its skin and leaves it there, outgrown and discarded, in favor of becoming a beautiful stranger?

Almost somnambulant, I allow Dr. S— to position me in front of an oval mirror on the wall. He stands behind me, putting his fingers on my temples, pulling the skin back and upward. "Look," he says. His voice is low and so near my ear that the little hairs on my neck rise.

The change in me, though subtle, is startling. My round, green eyes are now slightly uptilted, catlike, the eyes of an Italian movie star. I want what I see in the mirror, impulsively and fervently, conveniently forgetting that the previous procedure, which went awry and produced the bump in my lip, was also heralded to me by the doctor who performed it as revolutionary, the very latest in cosmetic surgery.

"If you do it today," Dr. S— says softly, "at the same time as your lip, I'll only charge you one thousand. Usually I charge sixteen hundred. I always give a break on multiple procedures." A beat passes. When I don't respond he says, "If you like, Alana can just throw it on your credit card."

Of the three plastic surgeons I've been to, Dr. S— was the first who did not raise his eyebrows upon noticing my age on my chart. He did not fix me with a quizzical look as I ticked off the procedures I'd already had: Lips. Nose. Cheekbones. Lips again. From that first consultation, I could see that with Dr. S—, nothing I asked for would be off-limits. It thrills me, the dizzy possibility of it. But it frightens me, too. Without the brakes of someone else's disapproval, real or imagined, to slow me, what procedures will I not undertake? How far will I go?

"What do you say, Hope?"

To refuse requires more assertiveness than I can muster. But is it only my innate passivity which is to blame for my inability to say no? In the heated intensity of this moment, my decision has taken on a mythical weight and importance. The stakes seem enormous: to risk losing Dr. S—'s favor; to languish forever in dreary girl-next-door-dom. "No!" I cry.

"What?" Dr. S—'s brown eyes are round with surprise.

"I mean, yes! Sorry. I meant yes. Let's do it." I'm relieved to hear the confident ring of a decision in my voice. Dr. S—'s approving smile warms me like the rush of love.

After a few minutes, during which Alix is presumably ushered

into one of the recovery rooms and a nurse tidies up the surgical
suite, I am invited to climb atop the freshly sheeted operating
table. My heart beats a tattoo in my chest. I have never been awake
for a surgery before. With the other procedures, I had only to endure those anxious moments before the intravenous needle was
slipped into my arm, and I drifted peacefully away. There are, I've
learned, different levels of unconsciousness. There is general anesthesia, the state closest to temporary induced death, in which the
patient's breathing must be assisted and the heart closely monitored. There is twilight sleep, in which local anesthesia is combined
with intravenous sedation; the patient has no memory of pain during the procedure, though he or she may, as I did during the nose
surgery, recall hearing things: bones crunching, a saw grinding
away. There is local anesthesia alone, in which only a specific area is
numbed. This is what Dr. S— will use on me today. It is supposed
to be the patient's choice, depending upon the amount of pain relief one wants, though today's procedure is minor enough that it
does not warrant more elaborate sedation. I have heard, however,
that some doctors prefer general anesthesia even when it is not
strictly needed, so that the patient is completely comatose and will
not involuntarily jerk or cry out during the procedure. It is easier to
work upon a motionless canvas.

There is another degree of sedation I have not mentioned, one
which cannot be found in any medical textbook but one which Dr.
S—, perhaps unknowingly, wholly administers to me: the semi-
conscious state I drift into upon entering any plastic surgeon's office, a state of such passive surrender that it rivals an injected
narcotic.

I recline on the operating table, giving myself up to the sterile
ministrations of the nurse, who drapes my body with a paper
sheet. And then—with odd appropriateness, the moment is heralded by a burst of classical music as someone switches on a
stereo—Dr. S— enters the room, wearing clean scrubs, his sterile
gloved hands held aloft. His coppery eyes above his surgical mask

are crinkly; he is smiling at me. To a soaring of violins, like a parody of surgery in a movie, he leans over me holding a large syringe full of anesthetic. At the needle's approach a gasp of dread escapes my lips, and to steady them he grips my chin in the fingers of his left hand, too hard, then with less force when he feels my lack of recoil. With my face tilted toward his, he could almost be leaning in for a kiss.

I close my eyes as the tiny sting erupts into a riotous burning: a thousand wasps assaulting the tender flesh inside my mouth. I moan again, a low, strange animal sound. The pain is endless, unbearable; how long will it go on? My eyes overflow; water pools coldly in my ear.

"I can tell those are real tears." Dr. S—'s voice is tender. "Not fakey tears. You know how? Because they came out of the inside corners of your eyes. Fake tears come out of the outside corners." He pauses, holding the empty syringe aloft so that the nurse can take it from him and replace it with a slender, steel-tipped scalpel. "Thanks, Jeanne." Then, to me: "That's how you can tell if an actress on television is really crying or not, from where her tears come out. I'll bet you didn't know that."

Numb now, my lip feels thick as bread dough. The nurse dabs at my mouth with squares of white gauze, which come away livid with my blood. I close my eyes again.

Vivaldi soars on the stereo. Dr. S—'s hands on my face are cool and dry in their latex gloves. His breath through the paper mask is faintly minty. I feel my muscles begin to loosen, shedding the tension of the morning. I am safe now, in his hands.

"This is the thing the other guy is terrified of doing." He means the other surgeon, Dr. R—, who inserted the strip of Gore-Tex which is now pushing its way out of my lower lip. Gore-Tex is a synthetic material commonly used to insulate winter coats. It was supposed to give my lip a luscious, full look. But instead of a pretty pout, I got this unsightly, infected lump. A cyst, I told my roommates.

Dr. S— did not ask me why I didn't go back to Dr. R—. I think Dr. S— imagines that there is no reason for anyone to ever go to any doctor other than himself. Because he didn't ask, I didn't have to endure the shame of explaining that I was too timid, too easily intimidated to complain to Dr. R— and demand that he fix my lip. It seemed not so much a surgical snafu as my own just reward, for continuing to undergo what my mother calls my self-mutilation. It was easier for me to find another surgeon than to assert myself with Dr. R—.

Dr. S—, I know, would never make me feel ashamed for wanting to change myself entirely. Knowing this, I feel a confidence in his office that I do not feel anywhere else, and am willing to put my whole trust in him.

"How are we doing?" he asks, his voice husky.

"Fine." It's an effort to work my numb lips. Does he, too, I wonder, feel the intensity of the moment? Does he enjoy my surrender as much as I do? "Doctor," I say, a whisper, a slurred prayer.

"Hmm?"

"If there was an earthquake right now, and the power went out . . ."

"What would happen to you?" Dr. S— finishes my thought.

"Yes."

"I wouldn't leave you."

I wouldn't leave you. This is what I need so much to know. If the ceiling collapsed, if he were hurt, if he had to stagger to attend my supine body, he would. No price is too high for this safety, this guarantee of attention. My money, my flesh and blood, my dignity: I would give it all. *Is this what love feels like,* I wonder, *this desire for complete supplication?* The sight of my blood on his gloves seems appropriate; I already know that love and pain are intertwined.

Music soars on the stereo. I could lie there forever, helpless and inert. Is it sick to wish that a surgery would never end? Feeling a tugging at my temple, I ask, "Did you already start the lift?"

"Start? We're almost done." Dr. S— chuckles softly, pleased. "I told you it was quick. Turn your head the other way now, that's a good girl."

My eyes flicker lazily. There is a small metal table beside me, draped in blue paper, a few inches from my face. Atop it I see several bloody surgical tools, scalpels of varying thickness. Casually I regard my own blood, unmoved. But what is that other thing, that narrow strip of pale skin from which sprouts short, stiff brownish hairs like a squirrel's? What is this bit of roadkill on the surgical tray?

My eyes strain to see the floor beneath the tray. There, on the white linoleum, strands of my own long hair lie splayed in a messy heap. With a jolt, it hits me: My skin. My hair. My own severed flesh on the tray.

"Doctor." My voice is a croak.

"Yes?"

What can I say, now that it is too late? Is it not my own fault for agreeing so rashly to this operation? It had not occurred to me— nor did Dr. S— tell me—that he would have to actually cut out and remove a piece of my scalp on each side. Is this the shortcut of the procedure, the thing that makes it state-of-the-art? Won't it scar? Will the scars show? With the buzz of panic and regret come the familiar condemning voices: *You brought this on yourself, by making another fatefully bad choice. If you are scarred and imperfect after this, it is your own fault.*

My breathing seems to halt. *Calm,* I tell myself, *calm, calm. Breathe. Don't have a panic attack now. What's done is done.*

"Are you all right?" Dr. S— asks.

"Yes." The lightness of my tone contains a shrug. It shocks me, that I can feel such terror, and speak so offhandedly. "It's just that I'm staring at a chunk of my scalp on your table."

Dr. S— must be concentrating too hard on his work to have heard me. After a beat, he seems to register what I've said. His staccato laugh pipes out, "Ha-ha!" It is too loud in the operating room. "Did you hear that, Jeanne? A chunk of her scalp. Beautiful *and* funny! I like that."

His laughter washes over me. *Beautiful, he thinks I'm beautiful.* I close my eyes, trying to recapture the feeling of ecstatic surrender, a feeling so fleeting, so quickly departed.

I tell myself, *You are the straw that he will spin into gold.*

I almost believe it.

CHAPTER 1

According to the dentist, I was a late eruptor. That explained why, he said, that at almost thirteen I still had eight baby teeth in my mouth. I wondered if that also explained why I did not yet have breasts or a period like the other girls in my class, many of whom had, over the past year, burst into sudden, startling beauty like hothouse flowers. It would be a good idea, the dentist said, to have the baby teeth pulled out before we moved. We were moving from Los Angeles to Hong Kong for a year so that my father, a banker, could fix the problems the bank had in its office there.

Chop suey, rickshaws, the Year of the Dragon. I scanned the encyclopedia, eager to start our adventure.

The Chinese character for choice is the same as the one for confusion: I would learn that in Hong Kong. Choice equals confusion. "What on earth will I *do* there?" my mother wailed. There would be servants: a maid, a cook, a driver. She would have no obligations to fill up her days. How would she keep herself afloat in all that free time?

Three weeks before we left, my mother took a bottle and a half of sleeping pills and washed them down with Jack Daniel's. I was in my room wrapping my glass animals in tissue paper, my mouth stuffed with gauze and still swollen from having the teeth pulled, when it happened. I was wrapping the animals carefully, saying good-bye to each one before folding it away. I wondered if they would look the same to me when I unwrapped them in a strange place.

"Troubleshooting" was what my father said he was going to do in the bank's Hong Kong office. Seeing my mother limp in his arms, I thought that it sounded much like what he did at home. I heard the scolding wail of the ambulance as it approached our house and wondered what he would tell the neighbors.

In the hospital waiting room, I pushed my tongue into the tender, fleshy holes in my mouth, tasting the metallic tang of my blood. Beside me on the hard, narrow couch, my father folded and refolded the crisp cotton Brooks Brothers handkerchief he always kept in his pocket. My father had carried handkerchiefs since he was a boy, when they were the only gift bestowed upon him each Christmas and every birthday by his wealthy parents. I wondered how he managed to feign fresh gratitude each time when unwrapping the small, starched squares, each one monogrammed identically in navy blue with his initials, CHH.

Someone had left a pack of cards on the waiting-room table. "Do you want to play?" I asked him. "Gin rummy? Go fish?"

My father's head jerked from side to side but he managed a tight smile.

When my mother came home from the hospital, she looked pale and repentant. The doctors had given her a vial of little blue pills to help her relax, and she spent the days before we left sleeping on a chaise longue in our backyard, soaking up the thin June sun.

"Mom!" Sometimes I would call her, but she wouldn't answer. My mother's face in sleep always wore a curious look of effort, a crease of concern between her brows, her eyes squeezed tightly

shut. "Mom!" I'd say again. Then, more sternly, "Mother!" And finally, her name—"Virginia!"—seeing how it felt to call her that.
I'd get up close and peer behind her sunglasses, at her eyeballs
rolling back and forth under the closed lids like ships tossed about
on wind-swept seas. At school we were reading a book about the
ancient Greeks, and someone was always being tossed about on
wind-swept seas.

By the time we left, my mother was beautiful again. Unlike me,
my mother was fair and soft and lovely. I was darker like my father
and bony, all angles. I searched my face for signs of her beauty like
Ulysses scouting for land.

Once we got to Hong Kong, we stayed at the Hilton for several
weeks while we waited for our apartment to be ready. Our adjoining hotel rooms were done all in livid purple—drapes, carpet,
bedspread—a color which turned my mother's stomach and ag-
gravated her claustrophobia. There was a large picture on the wall,
a vividly rendered close-up of the inside of a purple iris. My
mother said it looked just like a vulva. I wasn't sure which of a
woman's secret parts a vulva was, though I was certain I'd seen
one in my mother's *Joy of Sex,* the icky sixties version where the
women had hairy armpits. The problem of the vulva picture was
easily solved—my mother took a scarf from her suitcase and covered it—but the suffocating color of the room was inescapable.
My mother wrung her hands, wondering how on earth she would
be able to tolerate three weeks of purple poisoning. The color sup-
pressed her immune system, she said. I wondered if sleeping pills
and Jack Daniel's would not do more harm than a color, but I
didn't ask. I also didn't mention what I'd found beneath one of
the beds in my room: an improbably large pair of shiny black
satin ladies' underpants, a remnant of a previous guest, who had
perhaps discarded them in a moment of sensual abandon. I
pushed them further under the bed with a coat hanger, wondering
how passion could occur in such an ugly room.

Every day, while my father worked, my mother and I went out

to explore the city with the guidebook the bank gave to all expatri-
ate families. She called our daily expeditions "field trips." We wandered down tiny, curving alleys where the acrid smell of sweat
mixed with fishy cooking. There were stalls selling huge dragon
pots next to hundred-year-old eggs soaked in horse's urine; disem-
bodied pastel-colored nylon bra and panty sets swung on plastic
hangers. Phony designer handbags sported Louis Vuitton or
Chanel labels, sometimes both on the same bag, following a skewed
idea that if one label was good, two were better. On Man Wa Lane,
we had ink stamps made of chiseled marble with our names on
them in Mandarin Chinese characters.

"At least we *think* they're our names." My mother nudged me.
"That's what they're telling us. For all we know these things could
just as easily say 'F-you.'"

We stood in Buddhist temples, stifling in the July heat, mop-
ping our faces with tissues and inhaling tangy swirls of incense.
Outside the temple gates, beggars swarmed around us, offering for
our sympathy sickly infants, gangrenous limbs. They thrust their
hands out, and we tried to drop coins into their palms without
touching them.

"Leprosy," my mother hissed.

When we got back to the hotel she ordered me to stuff my
clothes in laundry bags and jump in the shower and *scrub*. She
didn't believe me when I told her what the guidebook said, that
you couldn't become a leper just by touching one. Casual contact,
as they called it, was safe. You had to live among lepers every day
for at least seven years to be infected. It took that long to catch
their disease and become one of them.

Our apartment, on the sixteenth floor of a building called Twin
Brook, overlooked Repulse Bay, which my mother immediately
nicknamed Repulsive Bay. With the apartment came Lena, a Filip-
ina, to be our cook and maid, and Lee, who didn't live in the apartment but showed up every morning to drive my father to work in a
big white Mercedes. The way our servants lived, we were told early
on, was to be of no concern to us. Lena's room was a closet-sized

cubicle barely large enough to contain her foldaway bed. Her shower was a lopped-off black hose. These pitiful conditions were supposedly superior to the way most Chinese in Hong Kong lived. Once, my father came downstairs early and heard Lee taking his shower using the black garden hose behind the groundskeeper's shed.

Although the name Twin Brook conjured some peaceful, bucolic scene, there was, in fact, no actual brook to be found except for the muddy water that ran in rivulets down the mountain behind the building when it rained. I spent hours looking for capuchin monkeys in the jungly overgrowth there. Even though my mother said there weren't any, I was sure I would find one if I looked hard enough.

At the end of July, we got up in the middle of the night to watch television, along with the rest of the world, as Lady Diana married Prince Charles. I shivered with anticipation as I watched her descend from the carriage, a sugary confection of a princess. Like me, she was starting a new life, full of possibilities. Outside our windows, a monsoon banged the shutters of our apartment. Everything was new, and seemed magical.

The last field trip my mother and I took before I started school was to the Central Market, a slaughterhouse in the middle of downtown Hong Kong. We rattled along on the Number 78 bus on winding Chung Gap Road, our knees banging together and then sliding apart with each hairpin turn. Stepping off the bus into the crush and swelter of Central, we stood for a moment blinking and disoriented in the bright sun. Like a gasping fish I gulped great breaths of the humid air, which always felt more like water than air in my lungs.

The Central Market was an enormous green-canopied structure that spanned several blocks. Inside it was dark, the canopies blocking out all sunlight. The scene was lit by harsh artificial lights like the set of a slasher movie. The dense, tangy-sweet smell of blood hung heavily in the stale air. I felt it constricting my lungs, invading my pores, clinging to my hair. The cement floor ran with so much blood that the men who worked there wore special shoes with six-inch wooden platform soles to keep their feet dry. My mother and I wore thin canvas sneakers that were first rimmed, then quickly soaked through with blood. On the floor was a water buffalo head, chopped off and discarded, its dead, glassy eyes staring. I could not get my breath. Gagging, I tugged at my mother's arm to go.

"What's your problem?" Her eyes flashed at me. "We just got here."

"Please, Mom," I pleaded. "I can't breathe. It smells like . . . death."

"It's an *experience*," she snapped. "It'll toughen us up. I know *I* didn't ride that God-forsaken bus all the way here for nothing."

Her face was flushed with the high color her cheeks had when she was excited. I put my cold hand on her arm and she flinched. "Please, Mom. Please, let's go."

"You go. I'm going to look around some more."

I went and sat on the steps of an empty building across the street. The building was covered with a rickety web of bamboo scaffolding upon which men in shorts and bare feet clambered like monkeys carrying buckets of cement with no harnesses or safety ropes at all. I was glad I'd borrowed my mother's huge Jackie O sunglasses so that no one could see the tears running down my cheeks. I tried to take deep, even breaths, but all I could manage were a few shuddering gasps. My head, deprived of oxygen, felt it was about to explode. Later I would learn to identify this feeling as a panic attack. Then, I thought I might be suffering a stroke. The blood on my shoes had started to dry, making my toes stick together. Why did my mother want to linger in there? What was wrong with her? The longer I sat there, the more my crying changed, from tears with no sound to no tears but a small hiccuping sound.

Finally my mother emerged, blinking in the bright sunlight. Relief surged through me as I stood up and waved wildly. She charged across the street, ignoring the cars honking at her. As she flopped down beside me, I saw that her face wore a radiance I hadn't seen for months.

"God, this place is *sick*ening," she said. "These people are subhuman."

I understood, then, what it was about this place that soothed her: She could see suffering that wasn't her own. She sat beside me, watching the scene through narrowed eyes, and I could tell she felt at peace. She didn't notice the flies gathering on our feet.

My father worked late into the evenings because, he said, that was what all the bankers did, though my mother said it was to avoid us. When she wasn't screaming at my father, my mother directed her frustration toward the Chinese. "They blow their noses on the *street!*" she'd yell. "They spit to appease some *throat* God." And what was that smell, that foul smell that constantly surrounded her? "Everyone here comes up to my nose," she said. "I'm always smelling filthy, greasy hair." She began to take three, four, even five showers a day. My mother had always been hypervigilant about her personal hygiene, but this was a bit much, even for her. She claimed it was the humidity that made her shower so often; she couldn't bear to have even a drop of sweat on her body.

My mother made a friend, Harriet Evans, another bank wife who lived in our building. Harriet reminded me of Zelda Fitzgerald, but without the glamor. My stomach tensed every time I saw Harriet, who seemed always to be in a state of hilarity that struck me as vaguely threatening, as though she might try to hug me and slap my face instead. My mother and Harriet took classes together at the American Club. First there was "Mah Jong, Anyone?" ("The allure of the game is that it can never truly be mastered, as claiming mastery over a thing opens the door to endless trouble," I read in her book.) There was a gemology class, with my mother squinting through a jeweler's loop at smoky topaz and aquamarine samples on our dining-room table. Then it was "Beginning Cantonese," from a book with chapters like "Catching a Flight" and "Dealing with a Demanding Boss." The cover of the book showed a young blonde woman smiling and shaking hands with a tall, handsome Chinese man holding a briefcase. My mother learned *yat, yih, saam, sei, ngh,* counting on her fingers, and *m'goi,* the word for thank you, and then she quit. There was only one word a Western woman really needed to understand, Harriet said, and that was *gwailo.* It meant "foreign she-devil." Soon my mother, too, swore she heard it everywhere she went, on the bus, in the market stalls, even in the halls and corners of our apartment.

I wondered whether my mother really enjoyed Harriet's company, or if she just liked the fact that Harriet was clearly crazier than she was. Harriet and her husband were what the other expatriates called "lifers." They had been in Hong Kong for five years, and before that Bangkok, and before that, Singapore. They might never go back home. Everyone knew Harriet had lost it, my mother said, when she'd made the sweet-and-sour turkey for Thanksgiving. Her husband's name was William, but they called him Wild Bill Evans of the Orient. At dinner parties he talked openly about the eleven-year-old Thai prostitutes and fire-hose massages in Bangkok, while Harriet showed how open-minded she was by shrieking with laughter and pouring more wine. She had filled their apartment with every Oriental artifact imaginable, brass storks and monkeywood fish and delicate jade trees and bronze Buddhas. She even boldly displayed a penis-shaped candle that Bill had brought back from Tokyo as a lark.

I knew about all this because my mother told me. She always talked to me like a best girlfriend, like we were the same age. "What would I do without you, sweet apple?" she'd say, and I would feel the hum of our special closeness. I'd think, *So what if my mother is a little nuts? Weren't most beautiful women crazy?* There was something darkly romantic about it: On television the deranged beauty either got away with murder or met a tragic end. In classic novels, beauty and insanity went hand in hand; every hero-ine who threw herself in front of a train was heartbreakingly lovely. Besides which, I believed that my mother's craziness was a temporary state, like snow blindness, something that overtook her from time to time but which she ultimately had control over. My mother had a gift for all-out abandon that I both admired and en-vied, for I knew it was lacking in me. Like my father, I plodded along, being good, obeying rules, being *safe*. My mother did what she wanted. She smoked and drank and lay in the sun until she burned. When my father once complained about our water bill, she said, "I'll take fifty showers a day if I fucking please." I longed to know so definitely what it was *I* wanted, the way she seemed to.

Years later, a college boyfriend would say to me, "Your mother is pretty, but you're beautiful," and I would be both shocked and thrilled at the possibility of this. As a child, my mother's beauty shone like a beacon of hope to me, absolving her of all fault. Once, looking through boxes in my grandmother's basement, I came across an old 1960s Harlequin romance upon which was sketched, I was sure, a picture of my mother: a swooning beauty with round blue eyes, pert nose, shapely mouth, and long hair the color of but-ter. When my father called her "Hey, Gorgeous," I knew all was well in our house.

My parents met when they were freshmen at the University of Washington. My mother had grown up in Seattle and my father came to college there from Los Angeles. His parents had wanted him to go to USC or UCLA. They had hoped he would marry one of the Hancock Park girls he had grown up with. But my father had, to his credit, a rebellious streak that would not be squashed. He chose his college and he chose his woman. It does not surprise me that my grandparents did not know what to make of this small, pretty, nervous woman who showed up on their door, engaged to their only son.

My father first saw my mother as she was walking away from him. She was wearing a slim pencil skirt with a slit and a kick pleat, and he fell in love with her shapely calves. He followed her to the bus stop on Laurelhurst Avenue. My mother had a psychology textbook pressed to her chest, and my father said to her, by way of introduction, "How's psych?" My mother, I imagine, surveyed him with the weary look she'd borrowed from Lana Turner. "Handy," she said. "If you like manipulating people."

Nothing about my father's appearance hinted that he was the son of a wealthy doctor from Los Angeles. His worn trenchcoat was too light for the weather and his khaki chinos had a hole in the knee. He had a facial tic that flared up when he was nervous, which he always was. Only his Beta Theta Pi pledge pin indicated to my mother that he was someone worth talking to. My mother did like manipulating people, and in hindsight her first words to my father were remarkably honest. She gave him what amounted to a warning about herself. Whether she intended them to do so or not, her words told him exactly what he could expect if he fell in love with her. Which of course, he did.

Later that day, my parents had their first date, at a café near campus. In the middle of their table was a simple glass ashtray, and as they sat there, my father starry-eyed and my mother less so, the ashtray spontaneously shattered into pieces, shards of glass narrowly missing my parents. My father pronounced it a sign, that he and my mother were destined for each other. Probably his face twitched earnestly as he said it. But my mother had read that it was common for certain types of inferior glass to break apart like that. "All it *really* means is that we're at a cheap dive!" she corrected him.

My father was already well-acquainted with the disappointment of people he loved. His father called economics, my father's college major, "common sense made difficult." He had expected that his only son, Clayton Hathaway, would become a doctor like himself. When my father was fifteen, he took a summer volunteer position at the hospital where my grandfather delivered babies. Even then my father was a big man, six-and-a-half feet tall. He always slouched, even when sitting, as if he were sorry for taking up so much space in the world. On my father's second day at the hospital, a patient about to be wheeled into surgery suddenly thrashed about, pulling out her IV so that blood squirted everywhere. My father turned white, then ran from the room. A candy striper found him, throwing up in a linen closet. From that day on, he only set foot in a hospital if it was absolutely necessary. My grandfather, on the other hand, loved the hospital so much that his will stated that his entire estate was to be donated to it when he died. My father never overcame this early humiliation. It colored his idea of who he was and what he deserved. Perhaps he received my mother's lukewarm affection with the same resigned gratitude with which he accepted the undue economy of the handkerchiefs from his parents.

Many of my parents' early dates were study dates, and my mother said that she liked to stare at the crease that formed in my father's brow as he leaned over *Econometric Theory*. One of the things that most attracted her to him, she said, was his capacity for devotion to something that gave him so much challenge and so little reward.

CHAPTER 2

The heavy click of the dead bolt reassures me as I turn my key in the lock that my roommates probably are not home. "Hello?" I call out cheerily, relieved when my voice rings hollowly, unanswered, through the empty rooms. In the living room I pause, listening, in case one of the girls might be in the shower. I gingerly touch at my lip, which is swollen, throbbing, and has a tiny black stitch in it but is, at last, bump-free. As I'd hoped, the apartment is silent and still, save for a flurry of dust particles caught in a slant of sunlight.

I moved into the apartment from my parents' house a few months ago, after my fourth surgery, when my mother told me that she would not allow her daughter's "self-mutilation" to occur under her roof. A few months previously, I had moved back to Los Angeles after finishing my master's degree in journalism at U.C. Berkeley. My gilt-framed diploma hung on the wall in my parents' home along with various other mounted and displayed achievements, my bachelor of arts degree from USC, dean's list certificates, a photo of myself giving a USC campus tour to a CEO. I had drifted into graduate school the same way I drifted everywhere in my life, according to what other people said I ought to be or do.

My mother had told me, since I was a teenager, that I should be the next Jane Pauley. There was no reason, she said, that a pretty girl like me could not achieve this pinnacle of broadcasting. When I pointed out that it perhaps took more than good looks to do that job, my mother added, unfazed, that I was also "a people person." It shocks me, now, how little my mother knew me. I was most definitely not a people person. Though I hid it well, I was staggeringly shy. I was in a sorority, but I was not at all social. I led campus tours, but suffered panic attacks before nearly every one. The idea of going up to someone and talking to them, let alone sticking a microphone in their face, was unthinkable.

I had long ago lost interest in academic subjects, my early talent for creative writing eclipsed by my intense fixation on my appearance. In college, I rarely stayed overnight in my dorm room because I couldn't bear the thought of anyone seeing me without the armor of my makeup. When I put on my face, I put on my self, my persona, along with the blush and eyeshadow. When I concealed the circles beneath my eyes, I hid a myriad of insecurities and self-doubts. As I exaggerated the border of my lips, I sketched the outline of a bubbly, vivacious, confident girl. It was an exhausting daily performance. At the end of each day I needed to be able to wash off the mask and let my guard down, alone, before mustering the energy for another day's effort. Like a flower burdened by too much nectar, I was wilting under the strain of having to look perfect.

Being accepted to Berkeley, like all my other achievements, was a hollow accolade. I waved the acceptance letter around to my parents and my boyfriend, Hart, of whose affection I was never sure, hoping for a shower of praise that would temporarily soak my parched self-confidence. As if poured into a sieve, the good feeling my shiny accomplishments gave me drained quickly away.

Being accepted and actually succeeding in graduate school were two very different things. No one was standing around waiting to cheer for me. In fact, they were disdainful of someone whose only ambition was to be a television anchorwoman. My blonde good looks and sunny demeanor did not score me any points among my fellow students or professors. USC was all about being rewarded for the outside; Berkeley was intensely intellectual. Whereas in high school and college I had never had to try very hard to get good grades, at Berkeley I found myself among students who were as motivated as I pretended to be, real journalists in the making, many of whom were paying their own way through school.

I sank. From the first week, going to graduate school was an exercise in humiliation. Each day I felt more acutely aware of my mediocrity, of the elaborate farce of my life. Because it was journalism school, each assignment involved heading out into the world and accosting people. It was excruciating. I felt that my professors saw through me, saw my lack of ambition and what a sham I was. During the first semester I nearly failed all my classes. One instructor, an award-winning newspaperwoman, told me in her office one day that I should not expect to coast along on my looks. Which, of course, was exactly what I intended to do, not because I was lazy or vain, but because I believed that my appearance was all I had to offer.

To compensate for the incompetence I felt in the classroom, I embarked on a series of small, brutal romantic victories. I had always been fickle when it came to boyfriends. Except for Hart, with whom I'd played a cat-and-mouse game, I picked up and dropped suitors like trying on clothes. One boyfriend called me "the ultimate Gemini." At Berkeley, my romantic dysfunction kicked into high gear. I dated a series of my classmates, none for longer than a few months. I was proud of my reputation as a female Lothario, someone who usually tired of men before they tired of me. There was one boyfriend, Craig, to whom I was particularly unkind. He would call and ask if he could come over, and I would say yes. Then five minutes later I'd change my mind and call him back and say, "Actually, I'd rather be alone." Then I'd call him yet again, telling him that it would be all right if he came over, but just for a little while and only if he brought me a pack of cigarettes. The more Craig tolerated my cruelty, the more cruel and selfish I became.

Looking back, I cannot recall ever telling my parents just how miserable I really was. I maintained a sunny façade in every phone call and visit, though I often sobbed in my car along the desolate stretch of Interstate 5 between San Francisco and Los Angeles, a six-hour drive I made often with my cat, Midnight. On one trip, Midnight jumped out at a rest stop and I could not find her. Thinking she had run off into the desert, abandoning me, I sat down on the back bumper of my Jeep and began to sob. I couldn't even take care of my cat, let alone myself. I must have looked quite a sight, mucus and tears smearing the grainy highway dust on my face. I got back in my car, feeling my heart would break, the image of Midnight as carrion flesh vivid in my mind. I put Billy Joel's "You May Be Right" in the cassette player and began to cry again. Turning around to rummage for a tissue behind my seat, I saw Midnight there, peacefully asleep on the floor.

I had kept in touch with my college boyfriend, Hart, who had broken my heart by moving to Tokyo after graduation to teach English. When he called me one night and asked if I would come spend Christmas with him, I jumped at not only the opportunity to see him but at what I saw as a chance to escape from my life. I knew it wasn't me Hart really missed: He was homesick, it was cold, and Tokyo was so expensive he'd had to get all his furniture from a garbage dump. But I told myself he couldn't live without me, hoping desperately that once I got there I would, one way or another, not leave. I would throw myself on Hart's mercy and be a girlfriend, something I figured I had more skill at than journalism.

The pressure of the upcoming trip eclipsed the pressure of my classes. If I was going to go to Tokyo to offer myself to Hart, I had to be irresistible. Certainly I wasn't good enough the way I was. In college, I remembered sitting in a restaurant with Hart when he said, "You and I look alike. We both have sort of wide noses." This comment devastated me, though it wasn't something I hadn't already thought myself, in the realm of, *If I could improve something about my appearance, what would it be?* I often stared at my face, thinking about what I would change. With so much at stake, this festering thought turned into full-blown obsession. I absolutely had to get my nose done before I went to Tokyo.

Over Thanksgiving break, in Los Angeles, I booked a consultation with Dr. William D—. On December 2nd, I underwent a tip rhinoplasty in his office. I paid for it with the Visa credit card my parents had given me in college. It cost eighteen hundred dollars. I wanted to have a more extensive rhinoplasty, but my card had a limit of three thousand dollars.

Three weeks to the day after my surgery, I got on a plane for Tokyo. My nose had not healed completely, and it bled often and without warning. It began to bleed on the plane, somewhere over the international date line. It trickled in the shower at Hart's apartment. It dripped onto Hart's chest when we made love. It left a livid trail in the snow at a mountain inn we visited. Ironically, the only thing Hart noticed about my nose was that it looked larger. It was still swollen.

In spite of my beseeching, Hart had no intention of letting me stay on with him. I would hang around his neck like an albatross, he said, a listless and expensive decoration. And he was right: I had lost all confidence in my ability to hold a conversation, let alone a job.

By the time I got back to California, my nose had more or less healed. I was back to bleeding invisibly again, on the inside.

Instead of cutting my losses, I soldiered on at Berkeley. The gap between what I felt like inside and who I pretended to be was so profound, I often had a sensation of not being in my body. I would be walking across campus and suddenly be seized with the fear that gravity would suddenly stop working and I would topple into the vast emptiness of the universe. I avoided open spaces, feeling that the sky itself would crush me with its weight. Instead I drove my car to the edge of campus, parking as close as I could to each class even if it meant getting a ticket. Often I sprinted from car to classroom, pretending I was late, when in fact I was seeking cover.

Not a single one of my classmates was aware of my suffering. Like a rubber action figure, I simulated daily feats of everyday life. No one knew that my pliable perfect skin hid hollow plastic parts.

The day of my graduation, I drank too much champagne, flirted with one of my professors, wore a frilly off-the-shoulder white silk dress, and felt like a failure. As far as I could see, there was only one option for me, and that was to move back to Los Angeles and wait for someone to tell me what to do with myself. I figured I would get my bearings, see what happened. I was very good at waiting, I thought. Wasn't my life itself just a waiting game, with a few manufactured distractions?

The problem was, the wheels of doubt and anxiety in my head would not stop turning. A nervous mind and a life of idleness are a volatile combination, as I suppose my mother knew before we went to Hong Kong. I was too vain, or just too afraid, to dull my unhappiness with alcohol or pills. Instead I went back to what I'd always done, which was to focus all my attention on the small, manageable terrain of my face.

And so I found myself in this apartment, the fourth in a quartet of roommates, all single young women in their mid-twenties. Each of us has our own bedroom; we share two bathrooms. Our apartment consists of the upstairs floor of an old house on King's Road, a building which, like so many in the area, bears traces of past grandeur, when it was a stately Spanish-revival home. The old wood floors of the apartment allow me to know the exact comings and goings of each roommate, depending on her particular footfall and choice of shoes. Hillary, an assistant at a record company, wears chunky platform wedges which clump noisily; Karen's demure accountant's pumps click with efficiency; Anita, a UCLA student, has a heavy tread that makes her sneakers squish as if mired in mud.

Every morning I lie in bed and listen to the three of them

getting ready for work, for school, for whatever business or engage-
ments their day may hold. Showers run; coffee perks; hangers skid
on coatracks as clothes are shuffled and selected. I listen to their
preparations with a sense of wonder. How are they able to go out
into the world each day, fresh and full of energy, instead of crip-
pled by fear and plagued by dragging lethargy? How is it that I
have lost the knack for everyday life? It can't be that hard; people
far less educated and capable and robust than I am do it every day.
And yet I can't imagine going to a job, even looking for a job. Not
only would I surely fail at my responsibilities, I can't make it
through the day without lying down on my bed to rest every few
hours. I'm a slave to this flattening fatigue.

By nine o'clock, with the final slam of the front door, my
roommates are gone. The apartment is silent. It is then that I
emerge from my room like a ghost to haunt the empty rooms. I
sample what's left of the other girls' morning rituals: I sip whatever
coffee is left in the pot, still warm; I smell lingering drafts of perfume, hairspray, deodorant, burned toast. I'll eat the crusts of
bread left on a plate by the sink, collecting crumbs with my finger-
tip. It feels comfortingly appropriate to me, this nibbling around
the edges of life.

They must wonder about me, the new girl, who mysteriously
doesn't work and whose days are unaccounted for. I'm polite, eva-
sive, elusive. I prefer to remain anonymous. I don't want the risks
and exposure of intimacy. I don't want anyone to expect anything
of me, for surely they will be disappointed. I don't want to be more
than a phantom roommate. On the few occasions when we see one
another, I deflect their friendly questions with the swift skill of a
judo expert. I feel, sometimes, as if I am from another planet, one
whose warlike customs make the simplest human gestures of
friendship seem threatening.

The only place I feel safe, truly safe, is inside my bedroom. My
affliction bears the earmarks of agoraphobia. Going out, I am
prone to panic. I feel under scrutiny. My legs threaten to buckle as

I cross the street. I imagine drivers staring at me, mocking me from within the safe sealed spheres of their cars. I'm terrified of fainting, of falling down, of losing control. I imagine people must notice the mechanical stiffness of my walk. I exist in a fog of nameless shame, feeling always as if I have done something inexcusably wrong, breached an etiquette, angered someone, or done something horribly embarrassing, which I'm unaware of but which is nonetheless entirely my fault. It's exhausting and unnerving. Even in the market, selecting a melon, I feel idiotic and out of place. I never meet anyone's eyes. I have to remind myself to breathe, to walk.

It frightens me, sometimes, how reclusive I've become.

Now, in my bedroom, I catch my reflection in one of the mirrors on my wall. I'm startled, for a moment, at my uplifted eyes. This happens, for a time, after any surgery. I'm bound to forget the change I've made to my appearance, and so the sight of myself is, for a time, unnerving. There is reassurance in the familiar, however disappointing. I get up close to the mirror now, turn my face from side to side. I like my new eyes, I decide. They do look somewhat exotic; they will look even more so with dark makeup, perhaps some kohl liner. I will experiment with them, play with them as with a new toy; it will keep me busy for a while. Have I turned myself into my very own Barbie doll?

The incisions in my scalp have begun to itch as the lidocaine wears off; I am afraid to touch the thick black surgical thread that Dr. S— stitched into my skin. Months later, I will be sitting in a restaurant with a man and absently reach up to scratch my scalp; my fingers will locate a wayward black stitch which somehow escaped removal. I will pull it through my skin like a loose thread on a hemline and, embarrassed, tuck it quickly into my napkin before my companion can see.

I am lulled by the familiar rhythm of my days, which vanish into one another like waves on sand. Solitude never bores me, a fact which I probably ought to find alarming but which I chock up to having been an only child, all those hours of playing by myself.

Sometimes I watch television, drawn to the stories of misery and betrayal unfolding on talk shows and soap operas. I am soothed by the emotional slaughter of these people. Watching them wail, scream, claw at one another like animals, I feel mild wonder and envy. It must be liberating to flaunt one's pain so flagrantly. To regurgitate it up to the world on a television sound stage, to purge oneself beneath the hot gaze of millions. Often, I'll encounter someone whose obsession rivals my own. There are the food phobics, the self-mutilators, the dime-a-dozen neat freaks. There was a man who had driven his wife and family away with his compulsive cleaning and straightening. He spent hours neatening the minute threads of fringe on his area rugs. He actually used a comb. He sat there, this man, miserable and bereft and completely helpless in the face of his compulsion. On another show, there was a woman so concerned with her appearance that she applied a full face of make-up not only each morning but every night before bed, just in case there might be some emergency in the night which would require her to see someone. Perhaps my obsession could benefit from such televised exposure. Maybe, caught like a deer in the bright studio lights, I might be shocked into my senses. I imagine the cloyingly sincere host, Rikki or Jerry or Jenny, posing a carefully scripted question: *At what point, Hope, did you lose yourself, and gain only your reflection?*

What would my life be like without this obsession? I've endured it so long it seems almost like a friend. What would I think about? How would I fill the endless hours of inertia? What did women like myself do, before there were these endless options for self-improvement? Others in history have had my sickness, I know; I search out articles, programs, any material I can get my hands on which relates to my obsession, hungry for facts that may illuminate my condition. I have become a veritable encyclopedia of facts relating to appearance issues. For example, it was only relatively recently that the definition of feminine beauty has included a slim build, full lips, a small nose, and straight silky hair. In the paintings of

Flemish masters, women lounged like plump, lazy felines, showing off pre-Raphaelite ringlets, generous noses, thin lips, and white skin. How does this ideal jibe with the *Baywatch* look? If one of the ladies of those oil paintings were alive today, she would be shocked to find herself considered fat, pasty, frizzy-haired, and unattractive. She would be sent to Jenny Craig and plied by her hairdresser with products to tame her curls. It is hard to fathom that the mere turn of an ankle was once considered the height of sexiness. Now we must have overinflated bosoms paired with girlishly thin bodies, a combination which is rarely handed out by nature. Was beauty always so complicated, requiring women to risk their health and well-being? Marilyn Monroe, it is said, was suffering at the end of her life from the painful effects of having liquid silicone injected into her breasts. In Victorian times, women had glass globes inserted beneath the skin of their breasts. Then again, that was the era when any mental distress a woman suffered was attributed to a wandering uterus and dubbed "hysteria." So I guess I can't blame my obsession on our times, Hollywood, the media, or even my mother, though I would certainly like to.

More interesting facts: Plastic surgery itself, I read, came into being as a specialty in the early part of the twentieth century as a means of reconstructing the obliterated faces and bodies of men who had gone to war. Before the eighteenth century, a woman's beauty was measured not by her physical appearance but by her virtue. A kindly heart held more appeal than a glossed lip. In the early nineteenth century, the French government, to combat falling birth rates, instituted a massive campaign geared toward women which emphasized "physical culture." It encouraged women to focus on the well-being and functions of their bodies, to fear germs and practice good hygiene, which heretofore had not been a focus of interest; in short, to focus on their physicality, ostensibly for their own health, though the true intention was to make of them more robust breeding stock. Before that time in history, I imagine that human courtship may have been more like that of the bird kingdom—the quiet, virtuous women like drab brown wrens, while the men paraded their brilliant plumage. Museums are full of paintings of foppish gentlemen, their cheeks rouged, wigs powdered, their shapely legs displayed in tights and tutu-like skirts. Louis the Fourteenth favored a stacked heel. Human babies, I've read, respond more animatedly to a symmetrical face dangled over their crib. This preference for symmetry extends to the animal world, the theory being that a creature with evenly proportioned body and limbs is less likely to contain within their DNA a genetic mutation or predisposition to weakness. It makes me laugh, to imagine a penguin eyeing the ratio of black to white on a potential mate.

I seek out and devour these factual tidbits in an effort to justify my own fixation. But how can I explain the collapse of the rest of my life? When did I lose the knack for friendship, for simple human interaction? It happened some time after high school, although I was never the type to have more than one or two close girlfriends. In elementary school I had a best friend named Alisa Forest. We spent endless hours in her room after school, watching the guppies in her fish tank breed and give birth and breed again in an endless, exhausting cycle. We considered ourselves fortunate to not be female guppies.

Alisa was a talented artist. We entertained ourselves by doing what we called makeovers. Alisa would sketch some hapless imaginary woman, unattractive in the extreme, with bulbous nose, witchy chin hairs, a moppish mane of hair. It was my job to dictate to Alisa which of the sketched woman's features could be improved and how, and Alisa then resketched the result according to my critique. Neither of us had any interest in Barbie dolls. We needed to create what we wanted from scratch. Poor Barbie, blamed for so many eating disorders and body-image woes. Curiously, she did not affect me that way. I was only interested in the degree to which I could alter her: I lopped off her hair, used Magic Markers to enlarge her lips and reshape her eyebrows. Beyond that, her rubbery face was too static to hold my interest. As for the makeovers, Alisa and I both found this exercise endlessly entertaining and profoundly satisfying, though looking back now I wonder whether it might have hinted at a gestating obsession on my part.

Alisa went on to become an accomplished artist. Is she happy, I wonder, having fulfilled her early promise? My world, unlike hers, has not expanded but rather contracted back to one alarmingly similar to those days in Alisa's room. I consider myself reasonably happy in a universe no larger than my bedroom, the solar center around which I revolve being my mirror. It's ridiculous, compulsive, how many times a day I look at myself. I have to keep checking, to make sure I'm still there. It's like checking for a pulse. It's a habit which reeks of vanity, and so carries the shame of that deadly sin; I would be loathe to admit my obsession to anyone.

But it isn't as simple as vanity. I do not swoon at the sight of myself. Sometimes, it is true, I do think I am attractive. It is what I always hope for. More often, though, my eye asserts itself upon some flaw, however small. And the most ironic thing is that those rare times when I do find myself lovely, I am overcome with despair. I look at the bounty of my face and see the fruitless waste of my life, my potential. So much effort focused on so unrewarding a cause. It is much more comfortable and reassuring to see myself as flawed, a work in progress. A work in progress does not have to make major life decisions or face painful truths, because there are other, smaller but more immediately pressing matters to attend to. In this way my life resembles a list of errands, the top five or so of which consist of things I want to change about my appearance. But instead of checking them off, as I surely should have done by now, and getting on with the bigger stuff, I endlessly shuffle variations of those first chores.

It's so complicated; I don't like to think about it. But what else do I have to think about? I find myself conducting my own little therapy sessions in my room:

Self: Have you always been so obsessed with beauty?

Me: I think so . . . when I was a little girl, I wanted to be Brooke Shields.

Self: Tell me about that.

Me: She was like a beautiful alien. Her beauty set her apart and made her special and unique the way I longed to be seen as special.

Behind that astonishing, preternatural beauty, I thought, were depths of pain and longing, waiting to be uncovered like treasure and healed with a lover's care. I desperately wanted to be discovered too, to be read with a lover's rapt attention; but without Brooke's beauty, who would care enough to discover me? I invented ways in which she and I were alike. I believed I could read, in the planes and angles of her face, the emotional geography of a loner. We were about the same age, she and I. Yet there was a worldliness in her direct unflinching stare, gazing out from movie posters and magazine pages. A bored, tragic bravery. As if she had endured a world of pain, and still she survived.

I was, perhaps, even more naïve than my mother in thinking that a pretty face was all I really needed in life. A prince's kiss and great beauty: These things would awaken me. My mother's dream for me, that I would become the next Jane Pauley—poised and together, and asking the tough questions while looking fantastic—required an effort I was not willing to make. Instead I drifted along in a fog of pleasant wistfulness, as foolish as Gretel toiling after a trail of bread crumbs.

I never believed what I'd told the first doctor, Dr. D—, that the only thing about myself I wanted to change was my nose. Even then I was thinking cheeks, lips, maybe breasts. But I did believe that, after I'd fixed these things about myself, I would be happy. I would emerge from beneath the bandages like a butterfly from a gauze cocoon and fly off into the world, free and full of confidence. But I was gravely wrong about that. I did not realize that my self and my appearance were two separate things, that I could not fix the former by tweaking the latter. A few millimeters subtracted from my nose or added to my lips did not change the inescapable fact that the person I saw in the mirror was still myself.

Inertia came quickly. However aimless I had been in college, and however unhappy I had been at Berkeley, there was nevertheless always something I had to do next: another class to take, an assignment to fulfill, my parents to please, a boyfriend to impress. With no plan laid out for me to follow, with no one to dazzle or disappoint, I was lost. With Dr. S— I found, once again, someone who would tell me what to do and who to be. There was a crucial difference, however, between Dr. S— and the other people upon whose opinion I had hung: He held a scalpel.

What made Dr. S— even more insidiously addicting was that his opinion of my beauty seemed as changeable as my own. Some days I was everything he wanted in a woman, physically at least; other times, he would compare me to a not-very-glamorous actress. When I went in for my first consultation with him, before we even discussed the bump in my lip, he suggested that I have my nose done. I told him I'd already had my nose made smaller, by Dr. D—. "Well, he certainly turned the tip up, didn't he?" Dr. S— said. I suspected that he intended his remark to send me into a flurry of dissatisfaction and regret that I'd ever gone to any other doctor. His comment offended me, too, because I had not asked his opinion, had I, on my nose? What right did he have to criticize it? He said, "If your nose was just a bit longer, it would improve your looks by seventy percent." It was then that I crumbled inside. *Seventy* percent? I thought. Was I *that* far from beautiful?

There was a well-known scientific study in which laboratory rats were taught to press a lever in order to get a food pellet. Some of the rats got a pellet every time they pressed the lever; others only got a pellet sometimes. The rats who discovered they could be sure of getting food whenever they wanted it soon felt secure enough to press the lever only when they were hungry. But the ones who got food sporadically became obsessed almost immediately with frantically pressing the lever again and again, desperate for their uncertain reward.

I was familiar with this study. I was an educated person. I could see its relevance to myself and Dr. S—. From that first consultation, I sensed that each visit to his office would be like gambling, with its heady uncertainty.

It wasn't long before my visits to his office were what I lived for. I needed them to provide me with human contact, excitement, the fulfillment I wasn't getting anywhere else in my life. It was a tall order, and I was frequently disappointed. I only felt alive when in his office, but I was vibrantly, heart-tinglingly alive. What workaday job, what office with its water cooler and ringing phones and tedium, I thought, could possibly equal that?

CHAPTER 3

A party at Bill and Harriet's apartment shook my mother from the torpor she had fallen into after being in Hong Kong for almost eight months. The afternoon of the party, she shopped for hours for something special to wear. We went together to Stanley Market. While my mother ducked in and out of shops, I wandered away from her, toward the edge of the market, past filthy chickens crammed in cages and eels wavering like black ribbons in tanks. I admired stacks of lotus fruit and bought a single red-orange clementine for good luck in honor of the Chinese New Year. I ate it as I walked, letting the peel fall around my feet, listening to the women haggling in angry-sounding Cantonese. My mother had said that the water trickling down the market streets carried diseases and could give you warts and hepatitis and who knew what else. I stepped carefully, avoiding murky puddles.

My mother wouldn't show me what she'd bought. When we got home she locked herself in her room to get ready, refusing to allow even my father inside. What grown-up, thrilling world was she escaping into, behind her door from beneath which wafted scents of bubble bath, Charlie perfume, hairspray?

"Ta-da!" At six-thirty my mother shot out of her room and raced down the hall like she'd been fired out of a cannon. "What do you think?" She twirled around before us. She was wearing a shockingly bright, bare jumpsuit, halter-backed, of vivid magenta silk. It barely covered her breasts, clearly braless beneath the thin fabric.

My father's face had frozen halfway between a smile and a grimace.

"What do you think?" she cried again. "Don't you like it? A girl has to compete around here to make a splash, you know." She began to do a sort of frantic, shimmying dance, her breasts jumping around wildly. As I gaped, one popped out, her nipple like one of the round ripe berries I'd seen at the market. "Oopsie!" My mother tucked it back beneath her jumpsuit, then continued to shimmy and shake. It struck me as the most terrifying thing I had ever seen, my mother's bare breast in our living room. I sat stock still on the couch, unable to move. For the first time, it struck me that perhaps my mother's craziness was not something she could summon at will and control, but something that took control over her.

The stiff grin stayed on my father's face as they headed out the door.

My parents returned to the apartment late that night with a great slamming of doors and shouting. Listening in my room, I gathered that my mother had drunk too much and done something embarrassing with Wild Bill. She was slurring her words, laughing and weeping at the same time. I could tell my father was very angry because he kept his voice especially low and steady. The angrier he got, the more still he became, like a large wave gathering force from unseen depths. Occasionally a word would distinguish itself: *Sick. Help. Crazy.*

After a while, I couldn't lie still any longer. My legs felt twitchy and light. I hopped out of bed. I had gotten a parakeet, Chopsticks, and as I pulled the towel off his cage, his small bright eyes blinked alert. I took him out of his cage and he balanced uncertainly on my finger. Chopsticks couldn't fly. His wings were clipped, and he'd always lived in a cage and didn't know how to live any other way. It frightened him to leave the safety of his small, barred world; as I stood on my bed, lifting him toward the ceiling fan, he scurried nervously down my arm to my shoulder. I grabbed him firmly with my other hand and, standing on my tip-toes, deposited him on one of the fan blades.

There. He was stuck. He clucked and scolded and bobbed as I turned the dial that controlled the fan's speed. Slowly, I increased the speed so that at first he hopped from blade to blade, squawking, then, when it became too fast for his tiny legs to keep up with, he fell to the floor in a tumble of feathers.

"Chopsticks. Here, birdy." He crouched on the floor, eyeing me with what I was sure was a small angry eye. God, what a horrible person I was. What kind of person tormented a poor bird? Carefully, smoothing down his ruffled feathers, I lifted him back into his cage.

Somehow, in the midst of my misadventure with Chopsticks, the shouting had stopped. The apartment was eerily silent.

After that night, my father and all his things stayed in the guest room. It seemed like I hardly saw him anymore.

Sometimes, during the day, I'd play detective, going into his room and inhaling the scent of him, his soap and the stale officey smell of his suits. In the bathroom I'd smell his aftershave and look at the leftover bubbles of his frothy pee in the toilet. He worked late every night, so my mother and I ate dinner together in front of the television, watching one of the American shows, like *Dynasty,* dubbed in Cantonese, laughing at the sharp, braying sounds coming out of Joan Collins's mouth. Sometimes my father would come home while I was doing my homework alone in the dining room. He looked exhausted, his face as gray as his suits, and though he made an effort to ask about my day, it seemed halfhearted. I always said "Fine" or "Great!" to let him off the hook. Once I was dissecting a frog for biology class, and he tried to help me, holding the rubbery skin open with tweezers. My eyes darted away as his shaky hands tore the yolky liver, ruining my good grade. I told him it was all right, and he let us both pretend that it was.

At school, I heard stories of expat kids who'd gotten island fever, the polite expression for losing one's mind in Hong Kong. There was the American boy who had jumped off his parents' balcony, impaling himself on a flagpole. There was the Swiss girl just a few years older than me who had shaved off first her eyebrows, then her hair, and been raped in a Wan Chai bar one night.

Most afternoons I spent at the apartment of my Indian friend, Dina. Dina's mother wore saris and made elaborate, colorful candles, which she sold in stores. I liked to lie on the platform bed that hung on brass chains from the ceiling in their living room, resting my head on the colorful pillows and inhaling their spicy, foreign aroma. Dina and I would feed each other sugary sweets she called chum-chums, pretending we were princesses in the Maharishi's court. I loved hearing her speak their language with her parents, like a small, private world only they belonged to. Maybe having their own language bonded them together. Was that the secret? If my mother and I chattered away in Dutch or Hindi, would we better understand each other?

At home, my mother spent more and more time in her room, listening to Helen Reddy records. I could sometimes hear her thin, reedy voice straining for the high notes. She continued to shower frequently, even on days when she didn't leave the apartment and thus expose herself to the humidity. It seemed to me that she had turned her unhappiness into a fervent desire to be clean. I'd press my ear to her bedroom door, listening to the rush of water and "This Masquerade." Sometimes she would wander around the apartment, her hair always wet, her skin wafting the scents of soap and pain.

Some days, the stillness of our apartment closed around me like a fist. The silence became a ringing in my ears. I would want to scream, to shout and scream until the ringing went away. One afternoon when Dina wasn't home and I had nothing to do, I stood on our balcony, looking over the edge until my stomach plummeted down and then sprang back into my throat. It reminded me of a game I used to play as a little girl, where I'd hold my breath until I passed out. I'd pull the air into my lungs and lie down on my bed and count, sometimes making it almost to one hundred. The trick was to fight the overwhelming natural urge to draw breath; it was thrilling, in a way, to try and measure the moment when consciousness failed and I fell into oblivion. There was a single instant that felt almost euphoric. But I'd stopped doing it long ago, afraid of being found sprawled and unattractive, the way my mother looked when she drank.

Standing on the balcony one afternoon, I thought about a lot of things. I thought about how I was sixteen floors up, on an island surrounded by the ocean, tens of thousands of miles from home. I thought about how my mother could do things, crazy, dangerous things, without worrying about the consequences. I, on the other hand, worried endlessly. I remembered that once, after my grandmother gave me a glass of cranberry juice with a splash of vodka in it, I had lain on my bed, paralyzed with the fear that I'd destroyed brain cells by drinking it. Alcohol could do that, I'd read. I agonized for hours, trying to think of things I might not remember, making little quizzes for myself, thinking I ought to eat some fish to rebuild my damaged brain circuitry. Standing on the balcony, I could see for the first time that worrying was pointless. I didn't want the burden of worry anymore. I didn't want to be the responsible one. It wasn't fair. I wanted oblivion. I wanted to be like my mother.

Pulling a great breath of air into my lungs, I closed my eyes and began to count.

Getting to twenty, no surprise, was easy. It made me feel powerful, denying myself something so vital. Twenty-seven, twenty-eight, twenty-nine . . . Closing my eyes made my other senses more acute. I heard the whoosh of traffic, the far-off shouts of beach-goers at Repulse Bay. Thirty-eight, thirty-nine . . . I began to wonder what would happen if I actually did it. Would I tumble off the balcony? Forty-one, forty-two, forty-three . . . I thought of the little boy who had fallen off his parents' balcony, how his mother had found him impaled on the flagpole. Fifty-four, fifty-five . . . It was more difficult than I remembered. The drumbeat of blood in my ears was deafening; a pattern of colors swirled before my closed eyelids. I could feel my face turning red, my cheeks puffed out like a chipmunk. Sixty-five, sixty-six . . . My fall might be soundless, unnoticed, insignificant. Would my mother look for me? Or would I be discovered by the groundskeeper, my broken body arousing no more interest or concern than a doll's?

With a great spluttering of air that was almost a sob, I spit my breath out and gulped the damp, hot air. Tears stung my eyes as I squeezed them shut. For an instant, I thought that throwing myself off the balcony might bring relief, quick and black. But I'd hesitated too long; the moment when I could have done it passed. I sank to the cool tile of the balcony, hugging my knees, at once grateful and ashamed.

Because my mother didn't go out much anymore, if I needed clothes or something for school, I had to go with Lena, our maid. Lena didn't speak English, and I think she pretended to speak even less than she did as an excuse for assuming the pleasant innocuous expression she always wore around us. We never spoke of my mother.

I'd wonder what Lena was thinking about. Her home in Manila? The family she'd left behind? She wasn't married and had no children. I guessed her age to be around forty. My mother said that Asian women bloomed early and wilted quickly. Had Lena ever been beautiful? If she caught me looking at her she would blink vigorously once or twice, as if startled by my attention. It must have been uncomfortable for her, living with all the tension in our apartment. Her domain was the kitchen, and sometimes I'd catch sight of her white uniform and brown face bobbing tentatively behind the beveled glass, not wanting to disturb whatever scene might be unfolding in the apartment. She rarely spoke to us, and never above a whisper, but I'd caught her once on the back stairway by the servant's entrance laughing and talking in loud animated Tagalog to another maid. Seeing me, she looked contrite, and I felt badly for having interrupted her.

At Stanley Market we walked in silence. Sometimes Lena would buy something at a food cart, suddenly coming to life in a torrent of gesturing and Cantonese. She'd raise her eyebrows at me to ask if I wanted some, a polite, pointless gesture since I always shook my head no, remembering how my mother said you took your life in your hands eating at those places. My shopping trips with Lena were an uncomfortable pantomime of master and servant. I'd point to the jeans and shirts and shoes I wanted, and she'd pay for them with the money my father gave her. I knew I could take advantage of this, buying too much, whatever I wanted. But her indifference defeated me.

Once, though, there was something so important that I decided I had to involve my mother. After a humiliating episode in gym class, in which I discovered I was the only girl still wearing an undershirt, I needed, immediately, to buy a bra. I refused to go with Lena on an errand so intimate in nature, so I walked down the hall and knocked hard on my mother's door. "Mother!" I called, allowing an edge of indignation to creep into my voice. Assuming I'd have to wake her up, I went in.

My mother was standing nude in front of her full-length mirror. Her body shocked me: her breasts droopy, her buttocks strangely deflated, her belly button a sad, startled O. Worst of all was the low, keening cry that came from her lips. It reminded me of a nature program I'd seen about elephants, the sound they make when one of their own is hurt. They form a circle around the one that's injured, and raise their elephant voices in mourning. But it was only my mother there, singing her own sad song to herself.

I froze, staring at her. It was a minute before she noticed me. When she did, her face abruptly twisted into a grimace. "Go away!" she shouted. "Beat it!"

I backed down the hall to my room and sat on my bed. I felt like the air had been punched out of me. Slowly, my shock turned to simmering rage. I imagined what I'd say to her. *Look how pathetic you are!* But when my mother came into my room an hour or so later, I couldn't find the words. She was wrapped in her robe; her hair was damp and fragrant.

"This place is really getting to me," she said.

She sat beside me and stroked my hair. I wanted to hate her, for yelling at me, for her absurd version of an apology, but the anger ebbed out of my body like something melting. "Hey, sweet apple," she said. It had been a long time since she'd called me that. We sat side by side on the bed and I watched the needle rise and fall on the record I was playing.

Suddenly my mother cocked her head to one side. "It's that song!" she cried, jumping up. "That song I always hear you play. I *love* that song!"

"Dancing Queen?" I was surprised she paid attention to the records I played.

"C'mon. Let's dance!" She pulled me to my feet. At first I felt self-conscious, stiff and jerky, though my mother didn't seem that way at all. I wondered if she'd taken one of her white pills, but she wasn't spacey. She was a good dancer, moving her arms and snaking her hips gracefully. Why didn't I know this about her? After a while I got into it too. We shimmied and swayed and bumped our hips together.

Dancing queen, young and sweet, only seventeen . . .

When the song ended, my mother lifted the needle and played it again, and many more times after that, until we were both past the point of exhaustion.

The only chore Lena refused to do was clean the birdcage. Maybe she considered this my job since Chopsticks was my pet, but her refusal struck me as both odd and annoying, since she did all the other maid things like clean the toilets and change the beds, and the birdcage, to my mind, wasn't any worse than those. Just pull out the pan, crumple up the newspaper, fold in a fresh piece, done. I knew it was my job, but because I resented having to do it, I sometimes let the cage go so long it stank.

One afternoon I was changing the cage on the kitchen counter, with all the windows thrown open. Chopsticks clung nervously to the top of his cage as I pulled out the pan. I wasn't worried about him flying away; not only were his wings clipped, he was terrified of freedom. Besides, I was fast.

I turned around to retrieve a section of the *South China Morning Post* to fold into the tray. When I turned back, my mother was standing in the doorway.

"Phew!" Her face scrunched into an exaggerated grimace. "How long has it been since you changed that poor thing's cage?"

I wanted to slap her. How dare she criticize how I took care of my bird? How dare she, when she didn't even take care of me?

I took a breath to compose myself. I didn't know what I was going to say, but it was going to be short, cutting, and as cruel as I could make it.

"Shit! Oh, shit, your bird!"

I turned around to see that Chopsticks had flown out the open bottom of his cage and landed in the open window. He sat very still on the sill. I had never seen him fly. I thought he didn't know how. But as we watched, he sailed through the window with a fluid natural grace that lasted several seconds. Then, as if remembering his own inability, he fluttered and fell downward, disappearing from view.

"Oh, God, your bird! Oh, no." In her immaculate Lanz nightgown, my mother clambered up onto the counter and peered out the window.

"Let him go, Mom," I said, and I meant it. He might starve to death in the wild, but at least he'd have a few days of freedom.

"It's my fault he got out," she said. "I distracted you. Look, I see him! He's on the ledge." With a sprightly ease I had never seen before, she ducked her body out the window and hopped onto the dirty ledge, several feet below.

"Mom!" I cried. "Mom, what are you doing!" This is it, I thought. My mother has decided to kill herself. There's no way she would risk such filth just to get a bird. Jumping up onto the counter, I stuck my head and an arm out the window. There wasn't room for both of us on the ledge, a concrete slab just a couple of feet wide; to come even part of the way out would surely knock her off. I reached my hand out as far as I could; I couldn't quite reach the back of her nightgown. A sickening, bleak terror twisted my stomach. "Mommy!" I screamed, something I hadn't called her for years.

The stench made me squeeze my eyes shut, and bile rose in my throat. The ledge smelled rank and acrid, like pigeon shit, like soggy wet rotten flesh and feathers. I forced my eyes open, sure that what I would see was my mother's thin form careening downward. Instead she was leaning toward Chopsticks, who was huddled in a corner.

"I've almost got him!" she cried.

Her hand straining for the bright feathers looked bony and fragile as a twig. There was nothing I could do to stop her from falling sixteen floors to the ground below. I lunged forward, crying out as the windowsill scraped skin from my shoulder. With the jolt of pain, something in me seemed to shatter—my pretend aloofness, the illusion that I could take care of myself. In her satin nightgown, with her hair whipped back and the endless sky behind her, my mother looked like one of the stained-glass angels in the chapel at school. I imagined her floating from me, drifting up and away.

"Mommy!" I cried, but my voice was small and thin, gurgly with tears. "Mommy, don't go! Mom!"

My mother swung around to face to me. "What?" she snapped. "Will you *stop* it? How can I concentrate with you blubbering?"

I jerked back as though she'd struck me.

My mother balanced on the outermost part of the ledge, arms out, hunkered down like a surfer. "I've almost got him," she called over her shoulder. "Hand me something, a ladle or something, to nudge him toward me."

She wasn't looking at me, so she didn't see that I didn't budge. The fear and anger I'd felt moments ago had hardened into something else, matter changing form. My eyes watching her felt very bright and hard, like a cheetah's, two bright pinpoints of vision. *Everyone knew she was unstable. A terrible, tragic accident. A daughter left alone.*

"Hope, quick! Give me something." She was impatient now.

I reached into a drawer and pulled out a wooden spoon. Focusing on the precise outline of her form against the white sky, I reached out as far as I could, stretching the spoon toward my mother's back. I managed a small but firm poke to the back of her gown. It wasn't quite enough to knock her off balance, but it startled her. As she glanced back at me, her eyes round and questioning, she took a little surprised half-step back. Her foot failed to find its place on the ledge, and she began to waver. I watched in slow motion, suffused with a complete calm. Suddenly my mother was a cartoon character, reeling backward, her arms pinwheeling comically. It wasn't until I saw her mouth form the familiar shape of my name, soundless, that I lunged forward, the spoon falling out of my grasp as our hands locked together. She swung back into balance, crouching, one arm wrapped around her knees and a cascade of blonde hair covering her face. Her body shook and heaved; she was crying. "Mom," I said, regret twisting my stomach. "Mom, I'm sorry. I'm sorry."

My mother flipped her hair back with a teenage abandon, and I saw she was laughing. "Holy shit!" she said. "Was that a close one, or what?"

Holding my hand to steady herself, she reached Chopsticks and passed him back through the window to me. In an instant she'd climbed back through herself and hopped down. She stood before me, grinning wildly.

"I *told* you I'd get him," she said.

She held out her arms to me. Her face was luminous, smoother and younger than I'd seen it in months. Her beauty startled me, filling me with warmth and longing the way it always did. Whatever dark force had occupied me moments before vanished, and hope split me like a sunrise. My mother had risked her life for me. Not exactly for me, but for something that was mine! She looked so enormously pleased with herself that, even though I didn't really want him, I clutched Chopsticks to my chest to show how much her heroism meant to me. His little bird heart beat hard under my finger, like my own rapid pulse. I put him in the cage. My mother was still holding out her arms, and for a moment we stood looking at each other, breathing hard. I moved to embrace her, but after a split second my mother's body stiffened and I felt her begin to pull away. But I held her anyway, squeezing too hard, wanting almost to hurt her, to feel the give of her bones against me. She was so thin that something made a cracking sound in her ribcage.

"Don't," she said, pushing me away. "I'm covered in bird poop." She went off to shower.

For some time after that day, my mother's bright moment of bravery lingered in my mind, vivid at first, then gradually fading until I wondered if I'd imagined it. When I tried to recall that day, it seemed elusive, like the green flash that supposedly occurs at the moment the sun sinks below the horizon, but is always missed when you blink.

As soon as school got out in June, my mother and I flew back to California and spent the rest of the summer with my mother's parents, who had moved some years ago from Seattle to the small

Northern California town of St. Helena. My father would join us in August, and we'd move back to Los Angeles. My father was going to get a big promotion at the bank and make lots of money, my mother said excitedly, his reward for a year of troubleshooting in the Hong Kong office. We were going to buy a house in Hancock Park, the exclusive area where my father's parents, the Hathaways, lived.

Meeting us at the San Francisco airport, I spotted my grandmother's face right away, scanning the crowd with an angry brow as if we might have duped her and were not really coming. Seeing my mother and me, her expression softened.

"My Lord!" Her strong hands held me at arm's length while she studied my face.

"What?" I asked, frightened.

"Your whole face has changed," she said sternly.

"Um, my teeth finally came in?"

"I see that," she said. "But your whole *face* has changed. You don't even look like the same girl."

"She's growing up, isn't she?" My mother swooped down, putting her face next to mine. "Isn't my girl just a *young lady?*"

As we wound our way up the Valley past snaking rows of vineyards, the vines heavy with fat, ripe grapes, my grandmother's words played in my mind. It was true, the gap between my front teeth had closed when my back molars had come in. But my teeth alone could not explain why people looked at me longer than they used to.

My grandmother lived on a hill above the town's modest country club, and I spent the long July days practicing my butterfly stroke and playing tennis. The three of us would sit around the pool under the mushroom-shaped plastic umbrellas while my grandmother filled us in on all the town scandals, whose husband was running around with who. At night, my mother and I occupied twin beds in the musty guest bedroom. I guessed I was happy. Three weeks ago, I'd bled for the first time. Patches of wiry hair had appeared under my arms, like scrubby brush on tundra. My body was becoming softer, less angular; I could look down and see two smallish mounds of flesh in my bikini top which my mother insisted on calling "breast buds." I looked down often. My long hair had gold streaks in it from the sun. My mother had become her old self again, cheerful and chatty. She'd helped me select a dazzling green bikini—my first—that rode high on my hips, and she told me to lie in the sun next to her so I wouldn't be so pasty. I thought she said "pastry," imagining the creamy white filling of an éclair. Lately, we were often misunderstanding each other.

I lolled by the pool in my new bikini, hoping that Dominic LaChappelle, the cutest boy in town, would stare at me. My mother nudged me when she saw him looking. "His family has a vineyard," she hissed to me. "They've got the big bucks." When this failed to motivate me, she took a more direct approach. "Go talk to him! What on earth are you waiting for?"

But I just sat dumbly on my towel, staring at the constellation of moles on my stomach.

"Oh, you're hopeless!" she cried. "Now you've lost your chance. You've got to be assertive with a man."

I buried myself in *Seventeen* magazine, searching for articles on Brooke Shields. "A Day in the Life of Brooke" had pictures of Brooke brushing her hair, jogging with a big smile on her face, even swinging upside down from a trapeze because "stretching the arms and legs tightens the waist!" Beneath a picture of Brooke removing her makeup with cold cream, the caption said, "Brooke keeps her strawberries-and-cream complexion in top shape with a daily regimen of cleansing and moisturization." I'd pestered my mother to buy all sorts of different soaps and creams and still my complexion remained pale as a moon rock. But for the first time, I had hope for myself. And the whole world, too, seemed to agree that I had potential. I liked the changes in my body, and the new attention I got, but it felt disorienting, too, as if my mind had scrambled. I'd be walking by the pool, lost in my imagination, and suddenly realize someone was staring at me. My body would seize up with self-consciousness, and I'd have to concentrate hard to keep my arms and legs from moving too stiffly.

It became harder and harder to lose myself in thought. My new creative writing journal, a gift from my English teacher in Hong Kong, who said that it would be a crime if I didn't keep on writing, lay blank and abandoned at the bottom of my suitcase. It was as if I'd been administered a highly addictive drug called Being Pretty, and it was slowly taking over my system, killing off all the other things I used to be interested in. I thought about my looks all the time, wondering constantly who was looking and, if they were, what did they see? A pretty girl? A homely, gangly girl? I thought maybe I could will myself beautiful by sheer force of my thoughts; I couldn't lapse in my vigilance even for a second because then I might tumble back into obscurity. It was kind of exhausting, trying to gauge people's reactions to me all the time. I had been more relaxed, maybe even happier, before I stopped being invisible, but what right did I have to turn my nose up at this new gift, for which I had wished for so long and hard? I had been tapped with a fairy godmother's wand; how could I not feel lucky?

At night, the sun sank low over the hills of the Valley, turning the sky a sudden, impenetrable black. I had never seen such a black sky. It looked velvety, rich, like something you could stuff in your mouth in handfuls, like devil's food cake. After dinner, when my grandfather had shuffled off to his study, my mother and grandmother and I sat around the living room in front of the old black-and-white television. As the two of them talked, I sat on the floor in front of my mother, who would weave my just-washed hair into a tight braid down my back. Listening to their female voices rising and falling, it seemed as though they were stitching together a private fabric of shared discontent, as if by pointing out what was wrong with everyone else might help them to know what was right with them. Their conversation took on a rhythm, punctuated by clucks and sighs, almost lulling. Once, my mother leaned over me

and said, "Wasn't that so, honey?" and, even though I didn't want
to agree with what she was saying about my father, I allowed her
hands tugging my hair to make a motion like nodding.

On television I watched a gymnastics competition, with young
girls in pretzel poses. They practiced with their coach, a man about
my father's age though much smaller in build. His hands were tender and attentive on the girls' bird-thin bodies. The way he caught
them, as each girl landed from some perilous jump or flip, made
my throat close up with longing.

At night, just before sleep, I lay in the complete mountain darkness like the darkness of deep space beside my mother. Listening to
her even breathing, I turned my mind back to the moment just before our hands locked on the window ledge, the moment when she
needed me more than I needed her. Thinking of this as I sank into
sleep, what filled me was exactly what I'd felt all those years ago
when I held my breath before passing out—a moment of weight-
less elation before blackness.

CHAPTER 4

My father's parents, Clayton and Eleanor Hathaway, weren't the richest people in Hancock Park. There were the Van de Kamps and the Ahmansons and the Bannings. But my grandfather was revered because he handled something of utmost importance to them, something more precious than their money: He delivered their babies.

As a child, several times a year, I was sent to spend the afternoon at my grandparents' house, a sort of goodwill offering on my father's part. My grandmother would pick me up at school. I loved seeing her silver Cadillac slide up to the curb, then hopping in and sinking into the heady smell of leather. She always played the radio on a lively, jazzy station. I'd watch her manicured fingernails, polished and shiny as the inside of an abalone shell, tapping the steering wheel. She always smelled impossibly sweet, like gardenias, or angels.

When my grandmother and I arrived at the house, a stately

white colonial, her maid, Louisa, would always fix me the same snack: a grilled cheese sandwich and Cheetos. My grandmother and I sat together while I ate, at the enormous mahogany dining-room table. My grandmother asked me questions about my day, but there was something forced and awkward in her inquiries, as if talking to a child made her uncomfortable. I tried to be engaging. Above our heads an ancient crystal chandelier tinkled faintly, like teeth chattering. The crunch of a Cheeto in my mouth seemed gargantuan.

When I'd finished, my grandmother retreated to her bedroom to nap and I was free to wander around. A very large house has, when it is empty, an air of holding its breath. My grandparents' house was quiet and dark. My father said they kept the curtains drawn so that the sun wouldn't fade the furniture. My mother said they kept the curtains drawn because someone always had a hangover. I suspected both were right. There was an elevator—it didn't work, my grandmother had converted it into a closet—and I found this unimaginably exciting. An elevator in your own house! I stood in the musty darkness, pushing the mother-of-pearl buttons and imagining I was going up or down.

My father's younger sister, Diane, still lived in her girlhood bedroom on the second floor. Diane suffered from an array of vague but never-ending physical ailments: stomach distress, fatigue, lightheadedness. She was usually home, but if she wasn't, I'd sneak into her room and look at the big unmade sleigh bed, the stack of Rolaids on the nightstand.

In my grandfather's study was a hinged globe on a stand that opened at the equator. Inside were glasses and a crystal decanter full of brandy. Shelves of medical books lined the walls, and under the bottom shelf of books were stacks of *Playboy* magazines. Sometimes I would open one to the centerfold, a soft-focus beauty caressing herself, and wonder if there was any chance I'd ever look like that. I'd pick up the novel *Endless Love,* which had been made into a movie I wasn't allowed to see, and flip to the sex scenes, like the one where the boy puts his mouth on the girl, down there, even though she's bleeding. I shivered, hoping I too would inspire such passion in someone. When I told my mother about the *Playboys*, she'd rolled her eyes. "You'd think he'd see enough of *that* at the hospital, wouldn't you?" she said.

If time permitted, I'd go outside and play in the summer kitchen, putting clay pots in the brick oven. There were seventeen fruit trees in their yard, including an ancient lime (which my grandfather called "the gin-and-tonic-tree") that bore fruits as large as fists. In the shade under the trees, I would collect small stones in the dirt, turning them over in my hand, looking for something precious.

My mother said the Hathaways didn't like her because she wasn't a society girl. But I suspected more: My mother needed to be fussed over to feel important, and the Hathaways were far too refined for fussing. Any excess of emotion had been bred out of them, like an overbright color dulled by many washings. When my mother arrived to meet them for the first time at eighteen, they did not offer her the fanfare she required. But then, who could have? The Hathaways probably fixed her with a diffident gaze while jiggling the ice in their highball glasses. Not only was this lukewarm reaction an insult to my mother, she didn't understand it. Her own family was volatile, vengeful, and unruly. My mother's brother had once tried to attack his wife on a dark road in Napa after she dragged him out of a bar, a story my mother told with a tinge of envy in her voice, as in, *See how much he loved her?* Such violent displays were normal, even expected, in my mother's family, the equivalent of a Hallmark card: They showed you cared. The Hathaways' reserve must have felt like a slap in the face to her.

My mother's resentment of them had become a kind of hobby to her, a small seed she nurtured over the years, turning it over and over in her hands until it was smooth and shiny as a pearl.

Other than those few afternoons, I saw my grandparents on holidays and at infrequent family dinners, which invariably included Hugh Bishop, a family friend, Hugh's wife Helen, and their two daughters.

My grandmother would always answer the door timidly, peering around as if it might be a stranger, even though she was expecting us.

"Hello, Eleanor," my father would say. "Hello, Clayton," to his father.

If it was a warm night, we'd eat dinner on the patio, and sometimes the soft smell of vodka on my grandmother's breath would drift across the table to me, mingling with the night-blooming jasmine. If my father's younger sister, Diane, was well, she would sit quietly at the table, sipping her ginger ale. My grandfather wore a pastel-colored button-down shirt with tiny monograms at the cuffs; his favorite tie was bright green with tiny martini glasses all over it. Everyone laughed when one of us girls begged a sip from her parents' cocktail and then scrunched up her face, pretending to hate it.

"They say drinking a little is good for your health," my father would attempt stiffly, trying for a joke.

"How would you know? You don't touch the stuff," said my grandfather, with a pointed look at his son's club soda.

After dinner the Bishop girls and I were released from the table to play in the yard. In the warm night air, I explored my grandmother's rose garden, which extended all the way along the back wall of their yard. I loved to read the little laminated cards my grandmother attached beneath each rosebush, naming the variety: Tipsy Imperial Concubine, Wee Jock, Champagne Cocktail, Sexy Rexy, and the one that made the girls and me laugh, Dick's Apricot Rambler.

My grandmother Hathaway tended her roses with a tenderness I never saw her apply elsewhere, not toward her children, her husband, or even the parties she planned with sterile, meticulous care, parties we'd later read about in the society pages of the *Los Angeles Times*. I longed to have her fold me in her arms, to feel her long fingers stroke my cheek with as much care as she used to graft an Heirloom rose. I wondered if I was the only one who noticed that when she left the table after dinner, she carried her plate through the kitchen and out the back door to her garden. I discovered her odd behavior one evening when, having excused myself to the bathroom, I saw her ghostly figure in the dusk, scraping the left-over lobster bisque and filet mignon into the soil around the rose bushes. She turned the dirt with her good silver fork, patting the ground as gently as a mother tucking her newborn into its crib.

I did not tell my mother about seeing my grandmother feeding her roses. I knew my mother would have ridiculed it, but I felt I understood why my grandmother did what she did. The roses were less frightening an object of affection than a person was. They received silently, asking nothing. Later, in the vibrancy of their blooms, my grandmother could see the reflection of her private care.

More fascinating, even, than my grandparents' house, was their country club, hidden at the end of a private drive behind gates in Bel Air. It was like going to another world. There was a library with dark-green fabric wallpaper, and black-and-white photographs of past club presidents and their families, the Drinkwaters and Griffiths and Jolicoeurs. Below the pictures were glass display cases full of ancient sports equipment, frayed croquet balls from the 1940s resting on velvet-lined shelves like the eggs of some rare ostrich, and old golf clubs, as delicate as whale ribs or finely carved Eskimo tools, labeled like extinct species: Lofters, Spoons, Niblicks, Cleeks, Brassies. A natural history museum of the very rich.

My mother called these dinners "command performances" or "an audience with the pope," meaning my grandfather, who always sat at the head of the table. But in spite of her protestations, she made sure that both she and I had something new to wear.

I sat quietly at the table beside my mother. I watched her fingers, folding and unfolding the starched napkin in her lap. I never spoke at these dinners. A child's place was to be seen and not heard.

I felt like I was at the axis of a spinning, moneyed galaxy. From other tables, I caught bursts of conversation:

". . . you don't mean the former pastor of St. John's, do you?"

". . . cream cheese, crab, and cocktail sauce. Delicious."

". . . telling Liz that Kate's going to wear *eggshell,* instead of white, if you can believe—"

". . . got a little *too close* to his parishioners . . ."

"Chili sauce, not cocktail. I ought to know, I used to cater."

"—everyone knows *white* dresses have always been the norm . . ."

". . . probably *enjoyed* it, actually, with a big, good-looking man like that."

Sometime in the middle of the meal, my grandfather asked my mother how she managed to stay thin, eating out as much as we did. My mother hated to cook, and my grandparents had referred often to the wasteful amount of money we spent on restaurant dinners.

I stiffened, praying my mother would not tell the truth. The truth would make her look like a fool.

"I always order something I don't like," my mother chirped breezily. "That way I won't eat it."

This was exactly the answer my grandfather wanted.

I felt myself hating her, suddenly, the way the Hathaways must have hated her. I cringed in my seat, steeling myself for the unpleasant scene that was sure to follow.

My mother's new dress was a frilly, white concoction with spaghetti straps and layer upon layer of sheer gauzy fabric falling to the floor. When I first saw her in it, I thought she looked like a fairy princess. Now, in the club's dining room, amid a sea of frosted hair and simple black cocktail dresses, she stood out like a grown-up parody of a teenager attending her junior prom.

My grandfather looked around the table to make sure everyone was watching him. He loved being the center of attention. When we arrived at the club, women flocked to him, his patients, laying their hands on his lapels and cooing with affection. I wondered if my grandmother ever became jealous; sipping her drink, she betrayed no sign.

My grandfather fixed my mother with a familiar devilish glint in his eyes, a look which I'd come to dread.

"I don't know about you," he said loudly, "but around here we call that the bimbo diet."

My mother's chest flushed red above the low neckline of her dress. Her freshly manicured hands fluttered at her hair. I felt a rush of sympathy for her, and longed to squeeze her hand in mine, to steady its nervous motion. I looked over at my father. His eyes were round and unblinking, his mouth slack. It was the same expression I'd seen once, in a miniaturized version, on eight-year-old Anna Bishop's face when, as a toddler, she'd slipped into the swimming pool without her water wings and Helen snatched her out—a look of wide-eyed, helpless terror.

My mother opened her mouth to speak, but the only sound that came out was a peal of tinkly laughter that was almost a shriek. It sounded as if she had a fishbone caught in her throat. A waiter rushed to refill her water glass.

"You're so funny, Clayton," she said. "And now, this bimbo has to pee."

It seemed to me as if the whole dining room were silent.

"C'mon, Hope," she said. "Accompany me to the little girls' room."

I rose from the table, my face burning.

Instead of heading to the bathroom, we went to the coat check where my mother retrieved her long wool princess coat from the uniformed black woman who worked there. Taking my arm, she marched us toward the vast sitting room which adjoined the dining room. Everyone was at dinner, so the room was ours. She chose a couch in front of the stone fireplace, so massive a person could have stood up in it, and she flopped down as if exhausted, patting the spot next to her. I sank into a musty cushion. My mother slipped off her heels and swung her legs up onto the couch, shaking out her coat like a matador's cape so that it settled over her.

"At least put your *feet* up," she scolded me. "We'll be here awhile."

I balanced my feet gingerly on the polished mahogany coffee table, hoping the leather soles wouldn't leave a mark.

"Do you think they're still talking about me?" my mother asked, not really a question.

I did not think they were talking about her. I thought of my plate with its half-eaten Dover sole and julienned carrots, cooling and congealing.

A waiter came by, and my mother ordered a Kahlúa and coffee for herself, "and a soda for Miss Brooke Shields here."

Eventually I stretched my legs out alongside hers on the couch, and we lay there like campfire girls on a cookout. My mother dozed, her contentment like fool's gold. Before the dinner, she had done my makeup. I always had to look better than the lackluster Bishop girls. "You're the *glam*orous one!" my mother gushed, stroking mascara on my lashes. I blinked my spidery eyes, hoping in vain she wouldn't start cranking out her stories about the Hathaways, stories in which, it was implied, they got their comeuppance. I had heard all these stories before, like the one about Helen and Hugh's first child, a boy, who had died shortly after birth. He was born with a heart defect, my mother said, and at the time there wasn't the technology to fix it. "Not even for Dr. *Hathaway's* friends' child," my mother said, a cruel edge of sarcasm in her voice. "And as you can imagine, *every* string was pulled." When my mother's meanness descended to these depths it made me cringe, because I didn't think she realized how cruel she was being, and also because her words so blatantly betrayed her own fear, how small she felt around the Hathaways, like a small snapping Shitzu, coiffed and perfumed, baring its tiny teeth as it backed away. There was a thin but very definite line between who my mother liked and who she hated, a line upon which I felt as if I, too, sometimes quaked precariously, for reasons I couldn't name. "Smile!" my mother said, and I obeyed as she blushed the apples of my cheeks, which ached with wanting to point out that if the Hathaways were as terrible as she said, then wasn't I bad too, because I was half them? Instead I pouted while my mother turned my lips into rosebuds, balancing the secret of our fragile tribe of two like a shard of glass on my tongue.

CHAPTER 5

Snapshot: a sunny Sunday afternoon, my senior year of high school. No picture was taken on that day, but if it had been it would look like this: the three of us, my mother, my father, and I, a perfect family trio, enjoying the day by our pool in Hancock Park.

It is unseasonably warm. Every day the few clouds that have gathered at night shred apart like cotton candy and the sky reeks blue, an artificial color like something drawn by Magic Marker. My mother is stretched out on the sun-warmed deck near the shallow end; I am lying on my stomach on a chaise lounge at the other end of the pool. My father swims laps. Both my mother and I wear bikinis. My high school's Winter Formal is approaching and, envisioning myself sleekly brown in my new red strapless dress, I reach back and undo the clasp of my bikini top to tan my back. Relaxing under the molten heat of the sun, I close my eyes.

My father finishes swimming his laps and gets out of the pool, hopping from foot to foot to shake the water from his ears. My father at forty is a good-looking man. He has aged better than my mother. Whereas in youth he was scrawny and gangly, with age he has filled out into a broad-shouldered, well-built man, with a thick head of wavy dark hair and blue eyes. He spreads his towel on the other chaise, beside mine; the lounge creaks under his weight as he flops onto it. I raise my head slightly, open one eye to smile at him. But he isn't looking at me. He is looking across the pool at my mother, who has abruptly gotten up, and strides into the house without a word. Just before she steps through the door, she gives him a look of such mysterious searing intensity that I shiver under the hot sun.

"What's with her?" I say, trying to be jokey, to make light of what I want to assume is just another of her mood swings. My father and I both ride the uncertain tides of my mother's emotional sea, although any acknowledgment of complicity between us is not allowed.

My father stares at the place where my mother had been as if she is still there. Something has changed, minutely, in the air between us. He says, in a stilted voice, "I think I'll go in."

My parents fight over the most trivial things; my mother's anger and unhappiness bubble up often and unexpectedly, like dinosaur bones in the nearby La Brea tar pits. I continue to lie outside by the pool, though my heart beats more rapidly now. Finally I gather up my towel and go inside.

Something is wrong. I feel it right away; my mother's rage hangs in the air like the stench of something rotten. Down the hall, from behind their door, I can hear my parents' animated voices. My father's, low and strained, is pleading, my mother's shrill and furious. Their door is closed, another sign that something is amiss, because my parents never close their door when they argue, nor do they confine their arguments to their room. Their battles are like installation art, a different vivid scene in each room.

Don't listen, I tell myself. *Don't bother.* I turn on the shower, one hand testing the water's temperature. There is a towel hanging on my bathroom door, but I tell myself I want a fresh one. Halfway down the hall to the linen closet, I freeze.

My mother is screaming.

"What the hell is going on between you two?" she shrieks. "Why did you sit next to her? Tempting you, in that little bikini! I know exactly what she's doing, and I know what you're thinking, don't think I don't!"

I know it, I knew it, yet still it takes a moment to realize: She is talking about me. I look down at my breasts in the bikini top, the flat terrain of my belly, and freeze with terror. *Dear God,* I think.

I cannot hear my father's panicked, protesting response. Whatever he says only seems to inflame my mother further.

"You're attracted to her, aren't you?" she wails. "Admit it! She's young and beautiful, and I'm not! I'm not an idiot, you know. Don't think I can't see what's going on here, right under my fucking nose!"

"I didn't sit by her, Virginia." My father's words are calm, measured, and perfectly clear. Does he know he's lying, or is sitting by me simply not worth defending? I want to barge into their room, smack him, to shake him until he acknowledges me. *I'm your daughter, for Christ's sake! What is wrong with sitting next to your own daughter!*

My mother's screaming changes: Her shrieks become wilder, like a baby's, long notes of rage punctuated by short stretches of silence during which she gets her breath. Through her screams I can hear my father's voice, protesting, soothing, beseeching.

I slink back down the hall to my bathroom, biting my lip to keep it from trembling. I peel off my bikini, avoiding the sight of myself in the mirror. I turn on the water, so hot I can hardly bear it. I push my face into the scalding spray, willing it to burn away what I've just heard, to sear the pain that has opened up inside me.

When I get out of the shower, I'm light-headed. My skin is red-purple, the color of a fresh welt. Holding very still, I listen. All is silent from behind my parents' door, save for the occasional rippling murmur of a television laugh track.

My head spins so much I can hardly stand up to dry myself. I lie down on my bed and watch the heat rise off my skin, plumes of steam lifting off my flesh.

Soldiers, I have heard, sometimes return home from war with pieces of shrapnel still in their bodies; they are astonished when its painless presence is revealed in an X-ray. As with every other drama, I know that the mottled fabric of our family will close seamlessly over this wound. I alone will betray its imperfect healing. My father may have dodged a bullet, but something jagged has lodged deep within me. No one will see it, and my parents in particular will never acknowledge it, but the damage inside can't be undone.

CHAPTER 6

In the back pages of *L.A. Today* magazine, a "Christian Cowgirl" can meet a "Presentable Widower in Good Shape." A "Mid-Western Beauty" named Allison offers "Sensual Massage with a Touch of Tantra, VIP's only." After Massage and before Personals is Dr. S—'s ad, a half page of promised perfection. Just as his office is full of young, attractive women—women like myself, I suppose—who do not look as if they need plastic surgery, so his ad features a black-and-white photograph of just such a woman, young, blonde, and slender. Her flawless face has a serene smile on it. Her head is tilted far back so that you can admire her perfect profile, and also because she is doing a back bend or some sort of vaguely gymnastic maneuver while wearing a clingy white T-shirt and panties. In letters tracing the curve of her upside-down stomach are the words *A New You!* It looks like a painful position to be in, but the woman's smile says otherwise, as if she is so satisfied with Dr. S—'s handiwork that even a difficult contortion feels effortless.

Sitting in his office, I realize that perhaps I am not so different from the lonely hearts looking for happiness in the classifieds. Is believing that a new nose or larger breasts will bring contentment any more credible than those other claims of instant gratification? Doesn't Dr. S——'s ad, with its offer of "A New You," hint at "Transformation Beyond the Physical?"

No one looks at each other in a plastic surgeon's waiting room. I always found this odd; shouldn't there be a sense of camaraderie, considering the risk each patient is undertaking? But I suppose it's not surprising. Plastic surgery is still something vaguely shameful, even in Los Angeles, something everyone wants to hear about but no one wants to admit they've done. It reeks not just of vanity but of cheating, having outsmarted or overpowered Mother Nature. Still, the degree of aloofness among the patients in Dr. S——'s waiting room is extreme. There is a definite competitive feeling, unspoken and unacknowledged, but undeniable. The first time I walked in the door and went to sit down on the sofa, there was something begrudging, almost hostile, in the non-look of the young woman who moved aside just slightly to make room for me. When I crossed my legs in her direction she flinched away as if I might scuff her aura. When the door opened and Dr. S——'s receptionist appeared to call someone in, all of us forgot our feigned nonchalance, our heads whipping toward her like springer spaniels flushing out an elusive pheasant. The patient whose turn it was bounded in, leaving the rest of us to simmer over our magazines.

I was instantly caught up in this invisible heated drama. Even though I have always detested cattiness in women, thinking myself above my mother's pettiness, I found myself imagining my superiority to the other patients in Dr. S——'s office. What were the chances that they had everything I did: an old-money family, an extensive education, brains, the whole shebang. I even found myself gloating silently over my debutante experience, which at the time had struck me as silly. My picture had been in the society pages of the *Los Angeles Times,* waltzing with my father, me in long white gown and him in white tie and tails, white gloves making his big hands look huge, like a clumsy mime. He spun me around the hotel ballroom, beneath a ceiling strung with tiny white lights meant to simulate a night sky strewn with stars, while my mother watched us from somewhere out of sight, beyond the hot white lights. I'd look around at the other women waiting to see Dr. S— and think, *You might be models or actresses, but I have breeding, for Christ's sake.*

But in the end my self-aggrandizing backfired, drawing me back to the same inevitable conclusion: If I was so perfect, then what was I doing at age twenty-three going from doctor to doctor, my big fat lack of confidence blowing the whole perfect picture to smithereens? I thought of how, when I first announced I was going to have the nose surgery, my mother disappeared into her bedroom and didn't emerge until a few hours later. She stood in my doorway, fresh from an emergency phone session with her latest therapist, James—who gave her, she enthused, "big bear hugs"—and announced that she could not understand why on earth her beautiful daughter was cutting herself up. I wanted to laugh, then, not at her dramatic description of my surgery, but because my mother never called me beautiful, unless there were people watching. In stores when I'd try on clothes my mother perched herself by the mirror outside the dressing room and insisted that I come out and twirl around. "Look at my beautiful daughter!" she'd exclaim to salesclerks, her effervescent praise uncorked by an audience. "Everything looks good on her. Isn't it just *sick*ening?"

I don't know whether it made it better or worse for my mother that the doctor I'd chosen for this first procedure was William D—. He was the only plastic surgeon I knew of. "Billy," as my family called him, was a colleague of my grandfather's as well as a longtime friend of my grandparents, who invited him to all their functions at the country club. I'd met him several times and I always thought it was funny that a man who focused on other people's appearances could himself be so unattractive, with crooked teeth and a long crooked nose. Billy was also my grandmother's doctor, one of her doctors. She was always seeing him to "have something re-moved," one of the pleasant euphemisms my family used. After-ward, she looked better, more rested, yet not in any way I could pin-point.

I prepared for my consultation with Dr. D— more exhaustively than I had for any final exam. I even brought a little powder com-pact in a shade slightly darker than my skin so that I could dust it down the sides of my nose to show him exactly how I wanted it slimmed. It took a little convincing, but not much, to get him to see what was wrong with my nose.

Once, years ago, I came across my mother reading this article in a beauty magazine with such rapt attention she didn't notice me. *The wrong lipstick color can make the difference between fatale and fatal.* For as long as I can recall, her bathroom cabinets have been full to bursting with products whose names promise "youth," "lift," "instant," "miracle." There may be gray in my mother's hair, but she has it colored to such perfection every three weeks that neither she nor anyone else will ever know. Maybe I wouldn't have desired her praise so much, if I hadn't known how much it meant to her to be beautiful.

It wasn't only my beauty that threatened her. Every time my fa-ther took a business trip, my mother quizzed him mercilessly upon his return as to what the stewardesses on his flight looked like. My father always claimed not to have noticed them, and he probably didn't, buried in bank papers. But with enough wheedling from my mother, he might cough up a detail or two, carefully unflatter-ing, like, "One of them had a big behind." This was all my mother needed to launch her accusations. How dare he have noticed them! As a child I missed my father when he was gone, which he fre-quently was, but the anticipation of his homecoming was tinged al-ways with dread for the predictable bloody ritual that went on.

I know that my mother, these days, considers herself much changed from that fragile and insecure woman. She jokes about getting older, even referring to herself as "an old fart." She thinks that therapy has brought her this inner peace, healing her from the inside out. It's a valid concept, except that my mother only stays with a particular therapist until he or she says something my mother doesn't want to hear about herself. Rose, her first therapist, lasted almost three months, until she told my mother she was childish. Soon my mother had abandoned Rose, claiming Rose had "a lesbian crush" on her.

If the wrong lipstick color can make the difference between fatale and fatal, what, then, would the wrong plastic surgery decision make? The difference between myself, familiar if disappointing, and someone I don't want to be? Do I even know a right decision from a wrong one, as I rush headlong to change my face and body?

Choosing Dr. S—, I know, is venturing into an area of risk I have not visited before. I do not know anything about him or his work; all I know is what I've gleaned from his glossy ad. And there is the fact that Dr. S— is not really a plastic surgeon; that is, he is not board certified to perform plastic surgery. He did not do a residency or complete special courses. He is a doctor who attended a few weekend courses. This is not illegal; many doctors are doing it, because there are no laws regulating who can and cannot hang out a shingle offering plastic surgery, and because it is for the most part a cash-only business, since elective procedures are not covered by insurance.

There is a large gilt-framed mirror on the wall of Dr. S—'s waiting room. I glance up often at my reflection as I sit there, hoping the other patients won't take my furtive self-scrutiny for vanity. Behind the glass partition, I can hear Dr. S— talking to his receptionist. "Tell Barbara that we can go ahead and liposuction her stomach again," he says, speaking of a female patient. "But remind her that she can eat faster than I can suck." His laugh is a short burst—*ha!*

I am looking into my own eyes in the mirror as I hear this. Inside, I both laugh and cringe. I am not blind to Dr. S—'s unethicalness. I know he is a phony, untrustworthy, passing himself off as someone he's not. But am I not also those things? I smooth a strand of hair from my cheek and hope I will be called in next. I wish I had not chosen a seat across from the mirror, which draws my gaze back again and again like a magnet. I look at myself quizzically, longingly, as one might look at a stranger. Who is that girl? Checking my reflection is a nervous habit I've always had; when I was small, before I was aware what hold beauty would have on me, I looked for myself in car windows, in pool surfaces, in store windows. It occurs to me now that perhaps I seek reassurance of a most primal sort: I need to make sure I am still there. Can it be that I do not feel substantial enough to even cast a reflection? Maybe my strangest and most secret fear is that I do not really exist; as if, between glances in the mirror, I might simply evaporate. It would explain why, just before I see myself, I always feel a blind, clutching terror that I might not be there. No Hope. No reflection. Nothing at all.

CHAPTER 7

The University of Southern California is a small oasis of rich kids in the ghetto. Fifteen minutes from Hancock Park on the Southbound Harbor Freeway, twenty-five with traffic. After the first day of registration it wasn't strange anymore to see the brand-new BMWs cruising around South Central Los Angeles. I kept the convertible top up on my car and stared straight ahead.

At home my closet was full of new sundresses for sorority rush. Rush was more brutally competitive than any beauty contest. The girls turned into piranhas in their sunflower-print dresses. I had never fared well in a competitive situation. My mother herself had dropped out of rush after the first day, but she told me that I, being "a people person," would fare better than she had. In my new dress, with a clip-on bow in my hair and my foundation melting in the August heat, I made the rounds with a herd of other girls to all the sorority houses. Immediately the group shifted into a makeshift caste system; I found myself among the girls who expected to pledge the best houses, the houses everyone wanted to be in because the girls were pretty and smart and popular. I had never been part of this elite crowd in high school, so the fact that I was so easily accepted into that group both thrilled and scared me. I went along with the cruel etiquette of rush: At the houses we didn't want to pledge, we asked to use the bathroom, so that we could primp for the good houses. Worse, even, than feeling my face grow shiny with sweat under the scrutiny of my potential sisters was the short walk between houses. The fraternity houses were on the other side of the same street, and the frat boys made a sport of rating the attractiveness of the rushing girls, holding up placards with numbers from one to ten. Terrified of the plunge my confidence would take if I saw a mediocre number directed at me, I hid in the pack of girls. It reminded me of Mutual of Omaha's *Wild Kingdom,* where a stampeding herd of wildebeests charges across the plains, the lions picking off those who straggled near the perimeter of the group.

I decided to pledge the Delta Gamma house, because the DG's seemed sunnier and less terrifyingly cool than the Thetas, who had, for their rush finale, performed a startlingly sexual leotard-clad number from *Cats.*

One afternoon a few months after starting college, I came home from class to find my mother sitting outside by our pool. Her eyes were closed and there was a book spread across her lap. I glanced at the cover—a bold primary-color rainbow, a couple of hearts. A self-help book. My mother's new therapist, Camille, was always recommending books to her: Reviving this, Reliving that, Reinventing the other.

"Hi, Mom." I plopped down onto the chaise next to hers.

"Hope!" My mother jumped in her chair, bringing a hand to her chest.

"Sorry. I didn't mean to startle you. What're you reading?"

My mother didn't speak so I looked for myself. *Hope and Healing for Survivors of Sexual Abuse,* it said; below, a line of smaller print announced: *A Workbook.*

I had just come from French class, where I'd had a test, and my mind, still in French mode, automatically translated it. *Workbook: le cartable.* My mother eyed me expectantly. I was supposed to say something, but what? Was this another of Camille's crazy ideas?

"I've been meaning to discuss this with you," she said.

My mind continued its absurd translation: *un cartable, des cartables. Avez-vous les cartables?* Sexual abuse: The words twisted sourly on my tongue, refusing to come out. "You don't mean . . . Grandpa?"

My mother nodded. "Camille says I have *all* the classic signs. She says it's why I've been so crazy all these years."

"When did he . . . I mean, what . . . Oh, shit, Mom! Are you *sure* about this? Do you *remember* things?"

"I don't remember anything specific *yet.*" My mother's tone was clipped, a bit impatient, as if she didn't appreciate being questioned. "But Camille says that's to be expected."

My eyes fell to her bare feet, her toes splayed apart with cotton balls. A bottle of mauve nail polish sat on the ground beside the chaise. I picked it up and turned it over to see the name of the shade: Plum Crazy. I felt like I'd stepped into a Fellini movie.

"We think it happened when he came back from the war," my mother said.

I thought of my grandfather, a timid and mild-mannered man, tending his koi carp and tying up his kiwi vines. The only thing I knew about my grandfather and the war were the seashells he'd brought home from some island in the South Pacific. As a little girl, I came across the shells in my grandparents' basement, boxes and boxes of delicately whorled and fluted creations. I'd thought it was romantic, picturing my grandfather as a handsome young man in his navy uniform, the way he looked in the picture on my grandmother's dresser, sending boxes of beautiful shells to his beloved. The shells rested on a layer of straw which, on closer inspection, turned out to be grass skirts. "Mom, look!" I called up the stairs to my mother. When she appeared I held a skirt to my hips and hula'd.

My mother wrinkled her face with distaste. "I'd forgotten all about those boxes. They stank to *high heaven* from the dead animals in the shells. And the skirts—they were full of *fleas!*" She blinked in the basement gloom, remembering. "Naturally, there was a fight when Mother wondered how he *got* those skirts."

Now, by our pool, my mother squinted off into the sunshine. Across the yard, a bird hopped around in the birdbath. "When Father came home from that ship he was so gaunt and sick, my brother and I ran from him, crying." Her voice had become hushed, with a little breathless catch, as if she were reliving the moment she'd told this story in Camille's office. "Mother wouldn't have anything to do with him," she whispered. *"Physically,* I mean."

Across the yard the little bird abruptly shook his feathers and took off, as though spooked. I thought of how my mother had, under the tutelage of various therapists, taken up and later abandoned interests in yoga, acupuncture, even a brief dabbling in white witchcraft, called Wicca. *Winter Solstice—Dance!* was still scrawled on our kitchen calendar.

"Is sexual abuse Camille's specialty?" I asked her now.

"Well . . ." My mother, I could tell, sensed a trap. "When she was a teenager, Camille was raped by her own brother." She leaned down to adjust a cotton ball between her toes. "So I sup*pose* that makes her sort of an expert in the field. But it's *much* more common than you might imagine."

"Right." I could barely contain a smirk of relief. My mother didn't really believe any of this; it was just another idea she was trying on.

"You know, Hope, a session or two with Camille might do *you* a lot of good, too."

"Excuse me?"

My mother looked at me over the top of her sunglasses. "You could figure out why you feel the need to stay in an abusive relationship."

She was referring to my boyfriend, Hart, with whom I was enjoying an intensely on-again, off-again relationship. "'Abusive relationship?' Please, Mom. He dropped me on the dance floor once. I skinned my elbow. Is that 'abuse'?"

"You said yourself he was like an addiction."

I had said that, it was true. I remembered my exact words, because I had thought about the situation for a long time. I'd said, "It's like I'm addicted to not knowing if he likes me or not."

Now my mother lunged forward on her chaise, her thin arms making me think of a praying mantis. "If he is an addiction then you must *treat* him like an addiction," she said. "And get started with a twelve-step program."

The skin above her bikini top, I noticed, was getting very, very red. "You're burning," I said.

"I don't care," she replied.

Two months later, in a lushly appointed dressing room of the Saks Fifth Avenue bridal salon, my mother and I engaged in a massive campaign to find me the right dress for my upcoming debutante ball. I'd already tried on more than a dozen at Neiman Marcus and Bullock's Wilshire. My mother had found something wrong with each one, some inferiority of design or fabric.

"For someone who claims to not care about 'high-society horseshit,'" I said to her, "you have very steep criteria for the perfect dress."

My mother looked at me sharply. "Do you want those other morons to show us up?"

I slid another dress from its hanger.

"We'll know it when we see it, won't we?" my mother sighed.

The selection of tulle and silk creations rustled stiffly like restive animals. Braced by cappuccinos, my mother and I worked our way through six promising candidates, my mother perched on an overstuffed pincushion of a stool while I tried on dresses.

I was halfway into a strapless white silk gown when my mother asked me, calmly and matter-of-factly, if my father had ever done "funny things" with me.

"It runs in families, you know," she said.

For a moment I couldn't speak. Then some necessary mechanism in my brain clicked, unlocking my tongue. "For Christ's sake, Mom," I spat.

"You're getting defensive, Hope. Which is why we need to discuss this in a neutral place."

I sucked my breath in sharply, as much to keep myself from cursing as to zip up the dress. *Ignore her,* I thought. As I stepped back a few feet to get a better look at myself in the mirror, I heard a tearing sound: One of my heels had caught on the dress's organdy underskirt. "Damn!" I cried, hopping around on one foot. "Shit, something just ripped under there."

"I really think a joint session with Camille wouldn't be such a bad idea." My mother tilted her head to one side, studying me. "What do you think about a cream or even a beige dress, as opposed to white?"

With a violent shrug, I unzipped the dress and shook it off, leaving it in a collapsed heap on the floor like a burst bubble. "How can you just switch topics like this, Mom? Do you hear what you're saying? How could you even *think* that Dad would do things like that? It's *sick,* is what it is. I don't know who's sicker, Camille for suggesting it or you for repeating it. Does she have you *brain-*washed? *Stop looking at me like that!*"

"Oh. You've finished," she said. "I just wanted to let you get all that off your chest. Camille said to expect this sort of reaction."

" 'Camille said?' *Camille said?*"

My mother sighed.

"Listen. Mom." I tried to get a hold of myself. "We're both tired. Okay? You've dropped a bomb on me here. Do you realize what you just said? It's . . . ludicrous. I know you don't believe it. I certainly don't."

"Don't you?"

"Let it go, Mom, will you? Just because Camille says something doesn't mean it's the truth."

My mother sat back and regarded me smugly. The dresses whispered on their hangers.

That night, thrashing sleeplessly in my bed, I couldn't get my mother's words out of my mind. "Funny things." It was bad enough that Camille had suggested such things about my grandfather. But my own *father?* Disgusting! Impossible. Insulting, really, was what it was. I'd report Camille. I'd call every state agency. Surely there must be someone, some board or committee, who dealt with such blatant cases of misleading a client. Maybe there were other clients she'd hoodwinked. I'd contact NBC News. I'd break the story. Yes! I really would be the next Jane Pauley. I'd . . .

Funny things. The idea crept in, spreading like a virus. Turning the thought every which way in my mind, even my own violent reaction to it began to seem suspect. What was that saying, about she who doth protest too much? I found myself raking through the settled dust of memory for anything out of the ordinary. As a little girl of four or so, I once pulled up my skirt in Sears, in front of an appliance salesman. Was it possible I was acting out some horrific private scenario? God, no. Ridiculous. But what about those times, all the times I rode around on my father's back, playing horse, on Saturday morning while my mother slept late—was there something more to that than I remembered, something I didn't *want* to remember? *No,* I thought, burying my face in the pillow. No. No. *No!*

As I teetered at last on the edge of unconsciousness, a thought appeared in my mind the way an animal shape forms in a cloud. That Sunday afternoon a few years previously, when my mother accused my father of favoring me. The memory stung. Suddenly, though, it was clear: My mother's reaction that day was not jealousy after all. It was her response to a perceived rekindling of perverse interest on my father's part. My God, she was trying to protect me!

My throat caught at the thought of it. I felt a rush of relief, then guilt. My Dad—how could I be so quick to suspect him? And yet, what other explanation was there for what happened that day? And wouldn't it explain, too, why my father had not touched me, not even a peck on the cheek, one single time since then?

In the morning I was trembling with fatigue and the over-whelming pull of this new idea. It was horrible, unthinkable, but appealing, too. In this version of events, I was not the villain. No one despised me. I wasn't "she." I was still a daughter, someone to be loved and protected, not suspected. Not rejected.

The thought swept me along. Over the next few days, it became less disturbing, the thought that my father had behaved inappro-priately toward me, though I could not remember anything even remotely specific. I stayed at the dorm, afraid that going home and seeing my father's familiar, friendly face would shatter the whole thing. I thought of nothing else. One afternoon on campus, when Hart came up behind me, I screamed and nearly jumped out of my skin.

"Jeez, what's with you lately?" he asked. "You're strung like a banjo."

I couldn't tell him what was with me, because it was too terrible to tell anyone.

That night, as I sat alone in my dorm room staring at my phi-losophy textbook with the white noise of rain outside my window, the phone rang.

"Hello, Hope?"

"Mom."

"I wanted to let you know that I set up a joint session for us with Camille this Thursday."

"Oh." I shivered. "Okay."

"I think we'll have a lot to talk about." Her voice sounded terse and ominous. I scribbled down Camille's address and we hung up. *Oh, my God*, I thought, *it's true. My mother knows things. She knows things that happened and she's going to tell me.* Was I ready for this?

Would I be able to handle such horrific revelations about my father? Oh God, oh God, oh God.

Time lurched forward, the days flipping over slowly. Finally Thursday came, and I arrived at Camille's building to find my mother's car already in the parking lot. We hadn't spoken since the phone call. I had imagined this scene a million times: My mother and I would fall into one another's arms, perhaps weep a little, overcome with relief at having overcome this terrible secret. Probably my mother had never willingly fallen into anyone's arms, not even my father's, but beneath the approving gaze of Camille, I was sure she'd make an exception. We'd talk at first about what each of us had done the previous week—small talk to ease us into the bigger stuff. I had gone to the final rehearsal for the ball. I'd tell my mother how I'd practiced my deep curtsy, and describe the ballroom ceiling, hung with tiny lights to give the effect of a night sky lit with stars. I would report proudly, too, that I was *seriously close* to giving Hart the heave-ho, and my mother and Camille would murmur how brave I was. Then the confessions would begin. My thoughts became blurry at this point, like the ambiguous soft-focus fade-out at the end of a movie.

Climbing the stairs to Camille's office, my legs were heavy. I walked into the waiting room and saw my mother sitting on the couch. Her expression made my stomach drop.

"Hello, Hope," she said icily.

It occurred to me that I could turn around and walk back out the door. But then Camille appeared, ushering us into her office. She was an anxious-looking woman with graying dark hair cut in a severe pageboy. She wore a gray suit and white blouse, with a bright floppy bow at her neck, a whimsical touch that looked forced on her. We went in, the door clicking closed behind us. The room looked like a shabby-chic living room, with a cloying disingenuous feel, as if its faux comfort was meant to trick you into a false sense of security. I sat down on an overstuffed denim couch by the window. My mother chose a poofy armchair at the very opposite end of the room, as if I might contaminate her. She sank into the fabric and crossed her arms, staring straight ahead.

Camille settled into her chair in front of us, crossing her legs primly. "Shall we begin?" she said.

I looked down, pretending to study the tight in-and-out weave of the beige sisal carpet.

"Hope." Camille said. "Would you like to start?"

"How can I start, when I don't know anything?"

The stillness of the room was suffocating. Somewhere above our heads, a clock ticked incessantly.

"Hope." Camille's voice was low. "Why don't you go ahead. Tell us."

"Tell you what?" I looked up at her. "What am I supposed to tell you?"

Camille blinked her eyes with the patient, satisfied air of a cow chewing its cud. I felt my face freeze. Hers, I realized, was the blueprint for the expression my mother's face had worn in the dressing room, when she had asked me if my father had done "funny things."

"This is all a mistake," I said, standing up. "I'm leaving."

Camille sprang to her feet, moving so that she stood between me and the door. "Now, Hope," she said. "Don't run away from this."

My mind, confused, soared back into French. *Qu'est-ce qu'elle dit? Pourquoi sommes-nous ici?* What is she saying? Why are we here? "You must be kidding, right? I don't believe this."

"I know it's difficult, but there's absolutely nothing to be ashamed of." Camille's voice was full of an eager, practiced soothing. "It's perfectly natural for a young girl to have certain responses, certain feelings, about the male figure in her life. It's just that some are appropriate, and some aren't."

"Responses? Feelings?" My voice soared into a shriek. "What the hell is going on here? Why don't you ask her about *her* feelings?" I looked over at my mother, who appeared to be simmering with some barely contained emotion. "What did she tell you? That I tried to seduce my father? Well? Mother?"

With a banshee cry my mother lunged out with her hand, sweeping a spider plant and the neat stack of psychology books on Camille's coffee table to the floor. She jumped up and stalked back and forth like a caged tiger in the limited space of the office. "I don't have to take this!" she shouted. "I won't listen to this little bitch accusing me of not being a good mother!" She stormed out the door, slamming it behind her so hard the windows rattled. A few seconds later she opened it, poked her head around and made a noise like a snarl at me, then slammed it again, twice.

We sat there, Camille and I, blinking at each other.

"Great," I said. "Nice work."

"We can try this again another time," Camille said. "We can—"

I got up and strode out the door.

In the parking lot I was surprised to find my mother leaning listlessly against her car, staring at the ground.

"Mom?"

Nothing.

"Mom!"

She looked up at me and blinked, a lost child awaiting instructions.

"Oh, shit, Mom. I'm going. See you later."

Pulling out of the parking lot, I looked in my rearview mirror. My mother was getting into her car slowly and stiffly.

On Sixth Street I stared straight ahead, focusing on the twists and turns of the road. Instead of getting on the freeway, I drove to my parents' house. Inside I strode down the hall to my parents' bedroom. I rifled in the drawer by my mother's bed until I found her credit card.

When I got back to the garage my mother was getting out of her car, with the same odd jerkiness, her expression glazed. "See ya," I said.

I drove down Wilshire to the department store, parked, and

strode purposefully through the large glass doors. The bright lights, the glass cases full of treasure like a pirate's loot, the endless shiny objects hummed around me, overwhelmingly. I wandered around for an hour or so, trying on lipsticks, pulling at clothes on racks, trying to recapture the feeling of angry purpose I'd had.

When I got home it was nearly six o'clock, time for dinner, but my mother was not in the kitchen. I saw the light on in my parents' room down the hall and went into my own room to read.

My father came home a short while later. I heard him call out, "Hello?" When no one answered, he came and poked his head in my room. "Where's your mother?"

I shrugged, to show I didn't know and, further, didn't care. I heard the heavy fall of his footsteps going down the hall and waited to see what would happen next.

A few minutes later I heard him coming back, moving quickly now, almost running, heading back to the kitchen.

"Dad?"

He didn't answer. I got up off my bed and headed toward my parents' room, my heart beating dully.

The sharp odor of scotch hit me at the door, as the supine image of my mother swam into view like an artist's soft-focus tableau. Bathed in the light of her Tiffany lamp, she lay on the perfectly made bed, in her blush-colored French terry Christian Dior bathrobe and matching slippers. Her hair was swept neatly back off her face, caught with a peach ribbon. Her feet were crossed at the ankles, and her hands rested atop each other on her chest. Her eyes were closed. She looked like a Byzantine saint in repose.

"Mom?"

Coming closer, I saw a letter tucked into the fold of her robe beneath her crossed hands. I recognized her Crane stationery with its swirling monogram.

"Mom!"

The bottle of Jack Daniel's was on the floor, empty. White capsules spilled across the carpet.

Everything wavered, then went still.

"Mom! Jesus Christ!"

My father came back into the room, carrying a glass of cloudy water. With his hand supporting her neck, he tried to hold the glass to my mother's slack lips.

"Dad, what are you doing? What is that?"

"Saltwater. To make her throw up."

"Christ, Dad. Don't give her that. Get her to the emergency room. Dad!" He seemed not to hear me, intent on trying to trickle some of the saltwater into my mother's slightly open mouth. It ran out the sides and down her neck, soaking into her robe. I snatched the letter away before it could get wet, noticing that my mother had tucked it into a matching envelope. If this was a suicide note, why had she used an envelope, as if she were writing a thank-you note or a dinner party invitation? I tossed it on the bed.

"Do you think she took that many pills?" my father said. "Maybe you're right. We should go to the hospital."

"I'll call an ambulance."

"No!" My father's tone was so panicked, I dropped the receiver. In a calmer voice he said, "No ambulance. Not at the house. The neighbors . . ."

My mother was mumbling about being sorry for something as he hoisted her unsteadily onto her feet, his arm hooked under her shoulders. I stood in the doorway watching them, chewing my lip. My father leaned down and said something into my mother's ear, and she moaned and rolled against him. I looked away, embarrassed, as if I'd caught them in an intimate moment. In an awkward embrace they lurched toward the door. My mother's head lolled against my father's chest and one of her feet in its slipper dragged behind her on the floor. It looked like they were doing a sloppy tango.

As they staggered down the hall, it hit me: This was the most physical contact I had ever seen between my parents. I hurried down the hall to the garage, where my father was folding my mother into the backseat of the car.

"Don't need an ambulance," my father was muttering. "Can manage just fine."

I thought of a day, years ago, when I had left the curtains open in my grandparents' living room. I had been playing with the crystal animals, and the sun shining through one caused a small plume of white smoke to rise from the carpet. I raced upstairs to my grandmother's bedroom, calling "Gram, there's a fire!" My grandmother rose up slowly, pushing aside her black satin sleep mask. "Call the fire department," she said. "But make sure you tell them to come with their sirens *off*, so the Malloys won't think anything's wrong."

"Do you want me to go with you?" I asked my father now.

"No. You stay here."

They left. I went back to my room, feeling jumpy and useless. After a moment I picked up the phone and dialed information for Camille's number. "This is an emergency," I told the woman who answered the exchange. "I need to speak to her right away."

A few long minutes later the phone rang and I lunged for it. "My mother went and tried to kill herself," I said to Camille. "She swallowed a bunch of pills and my father took her to the hospital."

"Oh, dear." There was a strange low, whirring noise in the background. "I see." Camille sounded out of breath. What was she doing, using a vibrator?

As the whirring slowed down, I recognized the distinct mechanical clicking of a bicycle chain. "Are you on a fucking *Exercycle?*" I said.

"I hear that you are upset, Hope." Camille's breath came in short quick bursts, like a poodle's. "Why don't we book a session for next week."

"I have a better idea." Holding the receiver as close as possible to my mouth, I shouted, *"Take your fucking session and shove it up your ass!"* I hurled the phone against my wall so hard a little indentation appeared below one of the flowers on my Laura Ashley wallpaper.

When the telephone receiver began its warning bleat, I did not put it back in its cradle. I have no idea how long I sat there—

minutes? hours?—in the same spot on my bed. After a while, I picked up a *Cosmopolitan* magazine from the pile on my night table and opened it, by chance, to an article titled "Fifty Ways to Drive Him Wild with Desire: Secrets the Pros Know." I closed it quickly, ashamed. It was entirely inappropriate to read a *Cosmopolitan* magazine while one's mother lay in the hospital, having washed down a fistful of sleeping pills with a chaser of scotch. But what *was* the right thing to do? Perhaps call a girlfriend, express dismay, seek comfort. I could think of a couple of friends who would act admirably in this situation, but I didn't feel like going through a pantomime of having to act upset, which I wasn't, and cry, which I didn't want to. It wasn't as if I didn't care, was it, just that I knew my mother was not in danger. She'd timed her maneuver to coincide with my father's six o'clock homecoming and, like the other times, probably hadn't taken enough pills before passing out to do any damage. It occurred to me that I could go and read the note my mother had written, but that, too, seemed unappealing.

What a joke, I thought. *What a fucking tiresome ordeal.* I was tired of this, was what I was. I looked down at the magazine in my lap. Opening it, I flipped through the pages to the sex article.

1. **Tease him with a feather.** *Right,* I thought. *Imagine trying to tickle Hart out of a drunken stupor with a feather. Fat chance.*
2. **Put some ice cubes in your mouth and kiss him all over.**
3. **Dress up like his fantasy of a secretary.**

Fifty of these? Jesus, you'd be exhausted by then. Were you supposed to do them all in a row? What a lot of horseshit, as my mother would say.

I tossed the magazine to the floor. My mother. What was she doing right now? Vomiting into a sterile pan? Explaining to some bleary-eyed psychiatry resident why her life wasn't worth living? I turned on the television. The noise and voices felt like needles. I turned it off. I lay down on my bed and hummed a little.

Around midnight my father came home.

"Why is the phone off the hook?" he demanded.

"I forgot," I said, ashamed. "I called Camille, and—"

"Exactly what did you say to your mother in Camille's office?"

I took a step back, as if he had struck me. "What? Nothing! God, nothing at all."

"That's not what your mother said." The light caught his glasses, making them go white.

"Dad—"

"To think that I would do those things," he said.

"Oh Dad, *no!*" The wind was knocked out of me, and instinctively I put my hands up to my face to make sure I was still there. "What did Mom say to you?"

"Never mind. I'm not going to glorify such trash by repeating it."

I wanted to throw my arms around his ankles and plead. But my father had turned away abruptly, and was striding down the hall toward their bedroom.

"Dad!" I called after him, addressing the retreating back of his business suit, a high, pin-striped gray wall. "Wait!"

My father closed the door. I heard the click of the lock.

I sank to my knees in the hall. Tears burned behind my eyes but would not come out. All feeling seemed to have ebbed out of my body. My heart ba-boomed in my chest like a hollow drum. I looked around me, blinking, at the bookcase with my high school yearbooks, my dog-eared copies of *Tom Jones* and *Candide*. I went back to my room and sat down on the bed, staring straight ahead until the tiny flowers on my wallpaper blurred. After a while I got under the covers without taking off my clothes and turned out the light. It wasn't cold, but I couldn't stop shaking.

Early the next morning, my father got up. I listened to the scrape of hangers in his closet, the rush of water, the low hum of his electric razor. I needed to use the bathroom and my tongue was thick and dry, but I couldn't make the necessary motions of getting out of bed. My mind darted around in the hard cage of my skull, but the rest of me was still. I realized my shoes were still on.

I heard footsteps coming down the hall, and in a moment the bobbing shadow of my father's head appeared in my doorway.

"Hope?"

I pretended to sleep, not wanting to continue any variation of last night's conversation.

My father cleared his throat loudly.

"Dad?" I pretended to stir as if I were just waking up.

"Hi." He managed a tight smile, his eye twitching violently. "I'm going to work now."

"Okay." Was I supposed to tell him to have a good day?

"I'm going to sue Camille," he said. "I think we have a pretty good case against her."

Sudden, overwhelming fatigue pushed down on me like a hand holding my head underwater. "Sure, why not," I said. "Sue her."

"One other thing."

"Yes?" I was surprised to feel hope stir in me, though feeble, that he would say something I needed to hear.

"Will you call your mother at the hospital? Just ask how she's doing? It's really the least you could do."

Somewhere inside me his words registered with a feeble bleat of pain. "Okay, Dad."

"Good." My father pulled a scrap of paper from his pocket and put it on my nightstand, where it floated liked a feather. "Here's the phone number."

I was so tired I could barely keep my eyes open.

He reached out awkwardly and patted the top of my head, twice. "I, uh, I cleaned up the bedroom, the pills and all." His voice had a forced jauntiness, as if he had discovered an unexpectedly optimistic ending to all this and was about to share it with me. "There's still a little brownish stain, but Marisa comes today; she'll get it. Not to worry." His hand patted absently at the breast pocket of his jacket. "Well. Okay, then. I'm off." He turned and took a few steps toward the door, then turned back again. "Oh, and Hope? If anyone asks, the neighbors or someone? Just tell them that your mother's out of town."

My mouth may have formed a response, but my mind had already escaped into sleep.

CHAPTER 8

Over lunch at a Greek restaurant, my mother's friend Sara raved about her latest face-lift. Having finished my degree at Berkeley, I had moved home to Los Angeles, where I had taken to tagging along with my mother on her social lunches. Sara was my mother's "westside friend," meaning that not only did Sara live in Pacific Palisades, but she was also nouveau riche, loud, and wore lots of jewelry—in short, the opposite of the reserved Hancock Park women in their linen and espadrilles. As Sara talked, I watched the light catch her aquamarine ring, which was the size of a small glacier; another, of smoky topaz, looked like it should go on over an evening glove. Jewelry, to my mother, was a telling measure of a person's social status; not how flashy and expensive it was, but rather what style and how one chose to wear it. An armload of bangles or a gaudy ring revealed a person's commonness just as tellingly as did the restaurants they chose to eat at. We once had neighbors who made my mother shudder with disgust every time they piled into their car for an evening of surf 'n' turf at Sizzler.

My mother always wore one "important piece" of jewelry, just like Jackie O. A single square-cut diamond dangling on a chain. A heart-shaped ruby cabochon ring with dazzling depths. When my father presented her with these pieces, her response was always the same: "Another bauble."

Over thimble-sized cups of espresso, Sara enthused about Dr. R—, her plastic surgeon. Sara was an attractive redhead with porcelain skin who did not, I thought, need plastic surgery, but perhaps it was because she'd had so much that she looked so youthful. Sara eagerly and unself-consciously spilled out the list of procedures she'd had: first face-lift at age forty; eyelid lift; forehead lift; tummy tuck; collagen in her lips and what she called her "marionette lines." During this last face-lift, just before the anesthesia took effect, Sara said that she told Dr. R— that it would be all right with her if, while she was out, he would just go ahead and fix anything else on her face or body that he happened to notice needed fixing. There did not appear to be anything about Sara's body that demanded improvement, but she hinted that her Chanel suit hid myriad imperfections.

In the ladies' room, I scribbled his name down on a cocktail napkin. I folded it and tucked it in my purse, my heart beating hard with hope. The pervasive emptiness I felt vanished; suddenly this lunch, this day, my whole life had meaning and worth.

Two weeks later, I sat in his Santa Monica office discussing my desire for higher cheekbones and a fuller upper lip, trying to sound convinced that A) I had put a lot of thought into this, and B) this was something I really wanted. While I had always pined for bigger lips, the cheekbone part was entirely random and impulsive. It was a matter of looking at my features and deciding what remained to be improved upon. I figured that if I was going to undergo the physical and emotional trauma of surgery, I might as well get more bang for my buck. At five thousand dollars, cheek implants were a pricey impulse. But I had acquired two more Visa cards, and I was as good at telling myself that I would never run out of money as I was at believing I was on a path toward something significant, that the surgeries were moving me closer to happiness. I didn't trust my intuition to steer me toward a good decision or away from a bad one. I was terrified of making any decision at all, and my fear paralyzed me. So instead of thinking, I jumped. It was so much easier to plunge feetfirst into a swimming pool, rather than stand there hopping from one foot to the other and wondering how cold the water was. That was what I told myself. Don't think, just jump.

Dr. R— was a short, plain man, nearly bald, the sort of man who accepts that he is not handsome and instead cultivates a certain look; in his case, that of an effete intellectual. The narrow oval lenses on his designer eyeglasses made his small gray eyes seem remote. He smirked at the mention of my mother's friend Sara. Both his manner and his appearance disappointed me. I had hoped to become infatuated. I could not read him, so I didn't know how to be. I tried affecting different personas: witty, slightly helpless, sort of tough. Nothing in his eyes told me I was charming or desirable. He stated rather than asked my age—"You're twenty-two"—with an upward jerk of his eyebrows which could have been amusement or surprise or condescension. I redoubled my efforts at being amusing and appealing, to no avail. Nothing increased my desperation like failure. Like Sheherazade, I felt as if my very life depended upon my ability to enthrall.

Sitting behind a desk that was as vast as he was diminutive, looking at me through his little glasses, I felt as if Dr. R— saw right through me, saw through my dog-and-pony show to the silly, shallow girl I was. I could have walked out of his office, could have found another surgeon. But I had already paid three hundred dollars for this consultation, and I was desperate.

On his desk was a photograph of his wife, a stunning woman.

Dr. R— suggested silicone implants for my cheeks and a combination of two procedures for my lips: The first, called a Y-to-V, would involve cutting the inside center part of my upper lip in a Y, then gathering and restitching the skin into a V to push it up into more of a pout. To plump out the sides, he recommended two thin strips of Gore-Tex, which would be channeled beneath the vermilion border of my lips via a tiny incision at each corner of my mouth. All of the scars, he said, would be hidden; besides which, the mouth healed faster than any other part of the body. The cheek implants, however, would be a more lengthy and complex procedure. There were several possible ways to insert them: through my lower eyelids, through incisions in my mouth, or from lifting a flap of skin in front of my ears. This last method, he said, was only suitable for women who were undergoing a face-lift at the same time as their cheek surgery, and there was no reason why I should have to suffer such obvious scars. The through-the-mouth method he did not favor either, as the implants had to be forced upward into the face and had, due to gravity, a tendency to slide back down a little, causing an asymmetrical result. He preferred the lower-eyelid route, which made me nearly faint with fear when he described it. He would cut just beneath each of my eyes, so that the scar would be concealed in my lower lash line. When he said *cut* and *eyes,* my head went light with panic. I wiped my wet palms on my jeans and hoped he didn't notice the dark spread of sweat beneath my armpits.

"I have a question for you, Hope," he said. "As to what sort of look you want. Would you prefer a Linda Evans or a Brigitte Bardot effect?"

I was surprised that he chose these rather outdated examples. I supposed they were each classic beauty types, but still, it made me wonder about the average age of his clientele. Was he accustomed to operating on such a young woman as myself? I decided it was pointless to worry about my age when it didn't seem to bother him at all. So, Bardot or Evans? I had seen pictures of Bardot in all her glory in the 1950s, as well as more recent ones in which she appeared startlingly aged. Linda Evans I remembered from *Dynasty*. I would have preferred that he offer me more youthful, contemporary examples of cheekbone structure. Still, it wasn't hard to make the decision.

"Brigitte Bardot," I said. "Definitely Bardot." It was a matter of deciding which of these women looked, in her prime, less like myself. Brigitte Bardot or Linda Evans? That was a no-brainer. It was the difference between being a sloe-eyed, platinum-haired French sex kitten and a bland all-American blonde with swimmer's shoulders and plump farm-girl cheeks, which I already was.

Everybody knows the Groucho Marx quip about not wanting to belong to any club that would have him as a member. As for myself, I did not want to look like anyone who looked at all like me. Offered a chance to dive headfirst into another persona, I didn't hesitate.

Because the operation would be extensive, I would need to be monitored closely for the first twenty-four hours after surgery. In lieu of a hospital stay, I chose a more Hollywood option: I would spend the night following surgery at a luxurious hotel-like facility which catered exclusively to post-op plastic surgery patients. It was expensive, fifteen hundred dollars a night, another charge slung effortlessly on my credit card. My credit was still flawless; I had paid every month on my old Visa card with the allowance my parents gave me at Berkeley. But the allowance had ended when I graduated, and I was now living entirely on credit.

My smile felt pasted on as I handed over my Visa to Dr. R—'s receptionist. As the card squeaked through the machine, I thought wryly, *A whole new me, accomplished in one swift magnetic swipe!* Was it supposed to be this easy to make such a drastic change in oneself, as easy as ordering something off a menu? And even though I could charge a new face as easily as ringing up a new dress at Saks, was I buying what I really wanted, transformation beyond the physical?

Merging into the late-day traffic on Wilshire Boulevard, these questions made my hands sweat and threaten to slip off the steering wheel. I began to panic, but my panic was always more endurable inside my car, where I felt safely cradled in a small space. Agoraphobia, I'd read, meant "fear of the marketplace," which I thought an extremely apt description of my condition, since I tended to panic in large supermarkets. Worse than the panic itself was the fear of public humiliation. I heard a story once about a woman who silently and politely choked to death at a restaurant because she was too embarrassed to draw attention to herself and create a scene. With the car doors locked and the windows up, I could panic in peace, without the worry of embarrassing myself. No one could see me cry behind my sunglasses, or look askance if I trembled, or hear me if I screamed.

I had been warned by Dr. R— that I would not like the sight of myself in the first few days following surgery. This caveat was even written in the post-op instructions: *Patient may wish to avoid mirrors for the first twenty-four to forty-eight hours following surgery.* While I didn't deliberately choose to ignore these instructions, I simply didn't think much about them. Or, if I did, I thought, *How bad could it be?* I had easily withstood the large T-shaped bandage on my face after the rhinoplasty, as well as the uncomfortable packing inside my nose and the purple-black bruises around my eyes. I had, in fact, marveled at their shifting color: violet, green, yellow, brown; who knew my skin could manifest such vibrant shades? It was miraculous, almost beautiful, like watching the shifting hues of a sunset.

My parents were out of town, but they knew that I was undergoing the surgery. They were both vehemently opposed to it, though my mother was the more verbal in her protests. "What on earth makes you want to do this to yourself?" she kept wailing. I had some inkling of just how devastated my parents were, but it hurt me to know how much I was hurting them, and I already felt so much guilt and foreboding about the surgery that I tried to block out their reaction as best I could.

Unlike the nose surgery, which was performed in Dr. D—'s office, this one would be at a free-standing surgical facility a few blocks from Dr. R—'s office. I took a taxi there. From the outside the building looked as unassuming as an office. But instead of desks and conference centers, inside there was sterile white operating room after operating room. I arrived there just before seven in the morning, as per instructions, and was led to a small, private pre-op room to undress and wait. The room was dimly lit and done in pastel shades. There was a needlepoint pillow of a rooster on the little bed and a print of sunflowers on the wall: a forced homeyness. As I slipped the thin cotton gown over my bra and panties and tucked my hair into the paper cap, I wondered how many other bleary-eyed patients quaked in their little rooms, alone with their last-minute fears, anticipation, and perhaps remorse.

In spite of the room's deliberately soothing palette, it felt like being in a holding cell. For a while I paced, my bare feet silent as a cat's on the floor. I felt like someone about to be marched to the death chamber, which I realized was an odd reaction since these were, after all, elective procedures. In the weeks leading up to the surgery I had done a good job of muffling the little messages of concern my conscience was sending me; now, in these last minutes, I was so nervous I wanted to put my fist through the pale peach wall, thinking that the pain of a broken hand would at least distract me. These were always the most difficult to endure, the last minutes before surgery, when you are still awake and aware of everything. I had brought a stuffed animal with me, a large white rabbit my mother had given me in college, when I was far too old for stuffed animals, but which I had nonetheless slept with every night since then. I called it my security rabbit. The rabbit's ears were lined with pink suede, its eyes two bright glass buttons. I brought it with me that morning not really for security, but because I hoped that the doctor and nurses would see me clutching this childish toy and offer me a child's greater portion of comfort. Holding it to my chest in the little room, I worried that it would seem a silly and contrived gesture, a worry which strikes me as ironic now, since the thought I ought to have fussed over was not whether I looked too old for a stuffed animal but whether I looked, and was, far too young to be undergoing such dramatic cosmetic procedures. How could a reputable surgeon operate in good conscience on such a young woman? I do not blame him or any of the others for decisions I made, but the question still nags at me.

I paced in the little pre-op room for almost an hour, wondering when the doctor was coming and chastising myself for using up all my energy being afraid when I should be using the time to center myself before surgery, to meditate or pray. I always said a short, stiff prayer in my head before surgery, accompanied by a fervent plea of apology to God for my otherwise appalling lack of attention toward Him. Pressing my face into the rabbit's soft ears, I rocked back and forth on the narrow bed. How could anyone relax in this room, knowing what was about to come next? The walls must have been rather thin, because twice I heard someone clearing their throat in the room beside mine, and a noise that could have been a cough or a fart. I tried to imagine the other patients, what they looked like, whether they were men or women. It occurred to me that some of them were probably here for corrective procedures, a hare-lip perhaps, or a burn victim, or to reconstruct a breast. Did it make them more certain of their decision and therefore less frightened than I was, I wondered, knowing they were here for something not just cosmetic but necessary? Was my fear really shame? Did it mean that I shouldn't go through with the procedure?

Another fifteen minutes passed. I had stopped pacing. I thought again of the other patients. How many had been called in to surgery, and how many were still buzzing with solitary anticipation in their little cells, like bees in a hive?

The door opened, and Dr. R— came in, wearing his green surgical scrubs and a paper cap.

"Good morning," he said. "How are we doing?"

"We—I mean *I,* am starving."

Dr. R— nodded. "I had scrambled eggs and bacon," he said.

This struck me as unnecessarily cruel, his boast of fullness in the face of my hunger. I could smell bacon and eggs on his breath, as well as coffee and, I imagined, toast with butter and jam. My mouth watered.

Dr. R— looked at the rabbit in my arms. "You won't be able to take your teddy bear into the operating room," he said.

"It's a rabbit," I said, knowing he didn't care.

Dr. R— took a purple felt-tip marker from the pocket of his scrubs. His little eyes examined my face from behind their trendy lenses. Perched up on top of his surgical cap were another pair of glasses, with tiny round magnifying lenses, which I imagined he must wear over his regular glasses during surgery. He held the pen aloft, sketching the air a few inches above my face. As he brought it closer I closed my eyes. I felt him begin to draw on my skin. It was an odd, almost ticklish sensation. I knew that doctors sometimes marked their patients before surgery, but it had not occurred to me that someone would do this to me. As he drew, tracing the lines where he would cut and stitch, making a map on my skin, I felt nauseated with panic. There was no backing out now. I was going through with it. My marked-up face made it real.

When Dr. R— tilted his head the light caught his glasses, making them go white. I held very still, like a good patient, my heart pummeling my chest so hard I was sure he could hear it. When he finished, he stood back, pleased with himself.

"See you in a few minutes, Holly," he said.

I sat there after he left, dumbstruck that he did not know my name. Maybe it was a simple mistake. But still, what if he didn't know, or even care, who I was?

I realized I had to pee. Suddenly, I was faced with a huge dilemma. If I went into the bathroom, there would likely be a mirror, and I would be faced with the sight of my drawn-upon face, which I imagined must resemble a vulgar Cubist sketch; a sight I most definitely did not want to see. I tried to never, ever think about that aspect of surgery, the blood and gore. I thought that the sight of my face would be too much for me to bear; it might send me running from the room, out into the street, screaming "No! No!" I thought, *You can leave now. You can still back out of this.* But why? What was the point of backing out of something I was bound to end up rescheduling anyway? Not because I had already paid for it, but because the anxiety and despair that propelled me here in the first place would not go away; they never fully went away, I only knew ways to pacify the painful longing inside me. The surgeries themselves were all-consuming, at least for a time— imagining what I would have done, who would do it, how I would look afterward—giving me something urgent to focus on instead of my pain. They made my inner turmoil more bearable by giving it a specific focus. *I'll feel fine after I have the tip of my nose fixed. The reason I'm so anxious and depressed and stuck is because I can't stand that little bump in my nose.* Did I believe it? Not fully, no, but it didn't matter whether I believed it or not. Just as my concerns focused on the physical, the outside of myself, so, too, I kept my thoughts about my motives carefully shallow as well. Backing out of this particular surgery would relieve the acute terror I felt right now, yes. But the constant, relentless tide of longing would return, as it always did, an ache that would push inside my chest until it became too intense to bear, driving me back to the operating room. I couldn't name this longing and I hadn't any idea how to overcome it. The longing existed, it seemed, both inside and outside of myself, a devouring beast. What easy escape was there from that?

You don't have to pee, I told myself. *It's just nerves. You haven't had anything to eat or drink since before midnight, so there can't be anything in you. Just don't think about it.*

When, at last, a nurse came to lead me to the operating room, I was numb with fear. I shuffled along after her, trying to remind myself to breathe. Down a seemingly long, narrow hall we went, turning the corner into a startlingly bright room, at the center of which was the slablike operating table, draped in blue sheets, with an enormous domed lamp overhead. Dr. R— was there, wearing his surgical mask, and about three or four other people, though I couldn't focus very well on how many people were there, or the machines bleeping and blinking, or the tray of glinting surgical tools. I climbed stiffly onto the table. Time seemed to be moving forward in spasms. My thoughts jangled like broken toys in my head, half-formed, mismatched. Just before I laid my head down I glanced at the floor, which was white linoleum, and thought: *Linoleum. Easy to clean.* Then the anesthesiologist slid the needle into my arm, and the world slipped away.

The operation for my cheeks and lips, I was told later, took three and a half hours. In order to decide which size and shape of cheek implant would best suit my face, Dr. R—, while I was asleep, inserted and removed a half dozen or so, fitting them into and then removing them again from my rubbery, inert skin as one might adjust or remove a foam shoulder pad from a jacket.

I awoke from surgery in a white room. Lying on a hospital gurney, swimming out of unconsciousness, my body shook violently from anesthesia. My legs jerked uncontrollably beneath the sheet, my knees banging the steel guard rails on either side.

"You want to see?"

A voice circled the air around my head, far away, like a hawk. I tried to turn my head, which was sunk into a pile of pillows. I was, I realized, tied at the waist to the bed by a kind of seat belt.

Slowly, I began to make out the room around me, which included a nurse standing beside me, her face a flesh-colored blur above her white uniform.

"You want to see your face?" she asked. She had a singsongy Asian accent.

Huh? Me? Now? I wanted to speak, but I couldn't seem to locate my mouth. My eyes would not focus, either; something thick and viscous had been smeared into them, something I could not blink away: an antibiotic ointment, perhaps, or something worse.

"You want to see? Huh? You see."

She had a strangely imperious voice, this nurse, not at all the voice of a caretaker. *No,* I tried to say. *No, I don't want to see. Not now.* I willed the words to come out of my mouth, but my lips would not move. I managed, somehow, to make a sort of frightened, bleating noise. As the nurse turned away, I knew to get a mirror, a spike of fear shot through me, in spite of the morphine. Did

I make, or had I made, some motion, a grunt or an involuntary nod, which the nurse took for assent? I would wonder about this later. Was it possible, unlikely as it seems since I could not speak, that I woke up asking to see myself, and the nurse was only obliging my request?

Stuck on my gurney, I could only wait for her to turn back to me. Just before she lowered the mirror over my face I thought, with a murky flash of hope, *It can't be that bad, can it? It can't be that bad if she wants to show me.*

"Here." The nurse held the mirror very close, so that my face filled the little oval. "Look," she said.

I focused as best I could on the image I saw in the mirror, which was most definitely not a face, not *my* face. It was something approximating a face: a pale, bloated jack-o'-lantern left too long on a porch, perhaps, or the face of a trauma victim, someone who had gone through the windshield of a car. It wasn't me.

I felt a kind of relief. In the mirror, I studied this atrocious sight. The mouth—not *my* mouth—was swelled up large as a purple fist, the face itself so big and shapeless that forehead seemed indistinguishable from chin. The eyes—here it seems the nurse held the mirror even closer—had the disconcerting appearance of being stitched shut, though I guessed that they were in fact just hugely swollen, with a line of black stitches underlining each one. What a face! What a sight! In my druggy state, I thought that it might not be a person after all but the face of a stuffed toy monkey I'd had as a child—a toy I detested for its handmade hideousness. The monkey's head was composed of an overstuffed white tube sock, with a thick black intaglio of cross-hatched stitches for eyes, a shapeless blot of red fabric for a mouth.

I jerked my arm out from beneath the blankets to touch this horrible, inhuman thing. Instead of fabric, my fingers touched skin, doughy and warm. And there were freckles! Just like my freckles. In the mirror I moved my hand across the giant bruised mouth, from which a bubble of blood pushed out, then burst. Wiping away the little red trail, my fingers moved across a little mole, distinctively star-shaped and ever so slightly raised up above the surface of the cheek.

My mole. On my cheek.

I was looking at my face.

A cry gurgled in my throat. The nurse continued to hold the mirror there for what seemed a long time. As in a nightmare, I could not move, could not turn away from the mutilated sight of myself. The cry became a weak wail, an animal's wounded keen. My body shook harder. The nurse and her mirror disappeared. Later it would occur to me how strange her enthusiasm was, how sadistic to insist that I see myself at that moment. There were too many drugs in my system to allow for all-out panic. Mercy was slipping back into unconsciousness.

The aftercare facility, in Century City, resembled a small, chic hotel. I lay in the vast mahogany bed, moaning whenever the Vicodin began to wear off, oozing blood and yellowish fluid onto the four-hundred-thread-count cotton percale sheets and immaculate European goose-down comforter. Outside my window, night fell like a hatchet. A soft-spoken blonde nurse with a Scandinavian accent appeared every so often like an angel from another world to adjust the drip on my IV. Soaring on a narcotic high, I asked her if she was one of the members of ABBA, come to take care of me. Hovering between waking and unconsciousness, I hummed "Mamma Mia" as she changed my dressings and tapped the slender tube in my arm. "Ah . . . haf . . . tuh . . . pee." When the nurse helped me to the bathroom, I asked her not to turn on the light. "You might fall," she said, flipping the switch. A huge mirror on the wall, just as I'd feared. *Why? Why?* My arms flew up to my face. Moaning under the harsh light, I tried to use the toilet without looking in the mirror. I felt like Frankenstein, reeling from the sight of his monstrous reconstructed face. *What have you done to yourself?* a voice wailed inside me. *What have you done?*

I had asked my parents to pick me up, forcing them into a yes by insisting that there was no other way for me to get home. The next morning, as I waited for them, I was even more swollen and bruised than I'd been right after surgery. I tried to be stoic, bracing myself for their reaction. When my father arrived alone, I was not surprised. I could not form my face into a smile and did not try to. My cheeks had become smooth, hard marble. The rearview mirror caught my father's eye twitching violently as he drove, though he didn't look directly at me. His face was the whitest I'd ever seen it.

I wanted to ask him what my mother was doing, what she would do. I was relieved when we got home and she was in her room with the door shut. A DO NOT DISTURB sign she'd taken from a hotel hung on the doorknob.

I went into my room and settled myself as comfortably as I could in my bed. A minute later, though, I had to get up again, to go throw up. As I leaned over the toilet, gagging and retching watery threads of mucus, I heard footsteps outside. I stood up, flushed, and pushed back my damp hair from my face. I opened the door. My mother was there.

"Ma . . ."

"Hope." My mother's mouth formed but did not speak my name, the way it had when she'd teetered on the window ledge in Hong Kong. She turned, disappearing around the corner. I could tell from her rapid footfalls that she was running down the hall. The door to her room slammed, and I could hear her saying, behind it, "Oh my God, oh my God," like a wail. I closed my door so I could not hear her and climbed back into bed, falling almost immediately into a comalike sleep.

Here is something you need to know about my mother: She always performed best in her maternal role when there was something wrong with me. Whether it be a bad haircut or a cold, she became an engine of motherly concern. She would bring me magazines, soup; she brushed my hair; she hovered. My physical weakness seemed to lower her emotional resistance. When I was little, I savored and exaggerated any sickness, so that I could stay home from school and be tended to by her. Her maternal temperature ran warmest when my body shuddered with chills. I would turn my fever-ravaged face to her, longing to feel her cool hand sculpt my cheek. Even as a teenager, when I would sometimes catch her studying me suspiciously, like a stranger, I could still depend on her affection when I was sickly. Whether it was flu or heartbreak, weakness made me both more compelling and less threatening. My mother became confident, more sure of herself and her role when I was ill. The boundaries between us as mother and child were clear and straightforward. I needed her. Healthy and robust, I knew that I became somehow frightening, even despicable, to her, though I didn't know exactly how. Damaged, though, I was a bird she could fold under her wing. It was the only time both she and I could be sure of her reaction to me.

But this was different. A case of the sniffles, too-short bangs, or a lousy boyfriend were manageable ailments. They did not threaten her own sense of security. This time, I had damaged the part of myself she both worshipped and feared: my appearance. It would be years before I understood that when my mother said, as she so often did, the words *my beautiful daughter,* she said them not for my benefit but for hers. My beauty was a shield she held up to the world to protect herself from scrutiny. When people swooned over me, her own failures and insecurities remained safely concealed. Even though a part of her hated me for being beautiful, for upstaging her, my mother was, in a sense, addicted to the idea of my beauty. And it went further than that: I kept up appearances for our whole small family. My parents had produced a single dazzling child; what greater achievement could be expected of them? Like a hood ornament, I represented to the world what was unique and important about us, distracting from what was damaged and hidden. Now, I had ripped off the mask of perfection and shown, most graphically, how terrified and fragile I was and, by extension, all of us were. For my mother, particularly, seeing my deepest, darkest insecurities made her think of her own.

I have heard that mother birds sometimes push their young out of the nest if they are sickly or deformed. As for my mother, she took one look at her disfigured offspring and fled the nest. She

checked herself into the Ritz-Carlton in Marina Del Rey and called
my father with explicit instructions that she would not come home
until I was gone.

When I called her on the phone, crying, and told her she was
abandoning me, she called it "tough love."

"Please," I begged her. "Please, please, I need you."

"I'm sorry," she kept saying, and I knew that she was.

"I'm sorry, Hope."

When my voice dissolved into unintelligible, choking wails, she
said, with something not unlike gentleness, "Crying like this can't
be good for you right now. I'm going to hang up," and she did.

That night, my father came into my room. He had made a tray for
me, a bowl of chicken noodle soup and a glass of Pepsi and some
saltines. A sick-person tray.

"I thought you might be able to eat some soup," he said, setting
the tray by my bed. He looked at my face, looked away, then forced
himself to look back again. His eye twitched, but he managed to
smile.

"Thanks, Dad." I struggled to sit up. "That sounds good."

My father stood there awkwardly, and I wondered what we
would say to each other. When he didn't speak, I said, with exaggerated enthusiasm, "Mm!" I brought the spoon to my bruised lips
and slurped noisily. Most of the soup missed my mouth, dribbling
down my chin to the front of my nightgown.

"Here." My father shook out the cloth napkin he had so carefully tucked under the spoon.

I dabbed at myself, then tried again. This time, I was able to
slide a few noodles into my mouth.

"Jeez," I said. "This is harder than I thought."

"Yeah," he said. "I'll bet."

"I'm fine really," I said, when he continued to stand there. "I'm
good. I won't choke to death or anything." Choking to death was

one of my father's worst fears. He had choked on a peanut as a child and had to be rushed to the hospital, where they put a tube down his throat. He always told my mother and I to take small bites. He had cut my steak for me until I was fourteen. Now I nodded my head up and down, to show how fine I was, how he didn't need to worry about me. I felt sorry for him, standing there, staring at his bruised-up daughter. He looked like he wanted to be excused.

"You didn't need to do this to yourself," he said quietly. "I don't know why you did this."

I looked down at the bodice of my nightgown, where a noodle had gotten stuck on a bit of lace trim. I retrieved it delicately, putting it on the tray. I searched for something to say that would make him leave the room. I didn't want to have this conversation. "Dad, please. It's a little late to be talking about this."

My father nodded; he was, after all, a sensible man. "True," he said. "But I still wish you hadn't done this to yourself."

"Okay, Dad." I was too tired to think of anything else to say. I thought it would be enough to let him know he'd been heard.

"Well, let me know if you need anything."

"Sure," I said.

"I have to go to work tomorrow," he said. "You'll be all right, won't you?"

"Of course, Dad. I'll be fine. I'll probably be up and about by the morning. I don't even need my painkillers."

"Okay."

When he left, I put the soup bowl back on the tray and put the tray on the floor. *I wish you hadn't done this to yourself.* I wish I hadn't done this to myself, either, Dad. I closed my eyes tight. I was afraid that if I cried, my tears would make the stitches loosen and the incisions sting.

Sometime in the middle of the night, I awoke parched. My face throbbed with heat. I sat up and reached for the glass by my bed. A few drops of Pepsi slid down my throat. I felt like I could die of thirst; my tongue was swollen.

The house was utterly silent. I swung my legs over the side of the bed, then heaved myself up. The room spun a little, then was still. I made my way slowly down the hall in the dark, trailing my hand on the wall for balance, heading for the beacon of light in the kitchen. When I came in, my father was standing at the counter with his back to me, pouring cereal into a bowl. He wore his charcoal-gray suit pants and a button-down shirt, so I knew it must have been about four-thirty in the morning. He had to get to work by five most mornings, so that he could be in touch with the bank's East Coast office. His jacket was draped over a chair. He didn't hear me come into the kitchen, my bare feet padding silently on the floor.

I didn't want to startle him. I said, very softly, "Dad?"

"Hopie! What are you doing out of bed? Are you okay?" In the dim kitchen light, in his dark pants and white shirt, he look bisected, severed neatly in half at the waist.

"I'm fine," I said. "I'm just so thirsty."

My father took a glass from the cupboard, filled it with water and handed it to me. I drained it, then another one. He watched me.

"There," I said. "That hit the spot. Thanks." For a moment we stood there, in the odd, ringing silence of the kitchen. "I guess I'll head back to bed," I said.

"Can you find your way back to your room in the dark?" he asked. "Are you all right to walk?"

"Sure, Dad. Don't worry."

"Why don't I get the flashlight. I don't want you to trip."

"It's okay, Dad. Really. I'm fine."

"No, no. Wait." He was fumbling in the kitchen drawers, shuffling through papers and dog leashes. "I know it's here," he mumbled. "I just had it the other night. Hold on."

"Really, Dad. Don't worry about it." I turned and started down the hall.

Suddenly his footsteps were behind me, then a burst of light.

"Ah-ha! I found it!"

In an instant he had sprinted ahead of me and, training the narrow beam on my feet, he walked backward, matching his pace to mine. We watched my feet, long and pale, ghostly white in the flashlight beam. My father stepped backward when I stepped forward, and I imagined we must look like some absurd cartoon in which one character is stalking another by mimicking their every move.

It occurred to me that either of us could flip on the light. But that would undermine the point he was making. So I stepped, more slowly and deliberately than necessary, letting my father direct the bright beam of light on each foot.

Finally we reached my room, and I crawled into bed, pulling the covers up around my neck. I was hot and shaking a little, a low post-op fever, maybe, or the anesthesia still wearing off. Directing the flashlight beam carefully at the floor, so it would be out of my eyes, my father leaned over me and put his palm on my forehead. "You're warm," he said. "Do you want a cool cloth for your forehead?"

"Yes. Thank you."

He went out of my room and down the hall, the light bobbing ahead of him. I heard him open the linen closet, walk to the bathroom, then water running. For a moment I thought, *My mother. Won't she hear us?* I felt a flash of panic. My father was taking a risk, doting this much attention on me. Then I remembered she wasn't home.

A moment later he was back, first the dancing beam of light, then the familiar tall silhouette. He lay the cloth across my forehead. He seemed to be looking at me, but a shadow fell across his eyes, so I couldn't be sure. "I'll leave this here for you," he said, switching off the flashlight, and I heard the clink as he set it on my night table. My eyes blinked in the abrupt absence of light, trying to make out where he was.

I wanted to tell him that it was not his small gestures of care-taking that meant a lot to me. It was the fact that he had not turned away from my face, gruesome as it was. And yet, how could I blame my mother for fleeing the sight of me? I thought of her, sleeping on starched white sheets in her hotel room, little bottles of shampoo and bars of soap lined up neatly, predictably. It occurred to me that the room she was in now was probably much like the room in which I had spent the previous night. My mother would be similarly doted upon and pampered, but could all that attention possibly relieve her pain? Did the sight of my face keep her from sleeping? What must it be like for a mother to see her daughter so battered, and how much worse to know that I had inflicted the damage upon myself? I had never spent much time thinking about how I might have hurt my mother, only the ways in which she had hurt me. I thought of her now, alone and suffering in her room as I had been last night. It occurred to me that we suffered alike in so many ways.

My father pulled the covers awkwardly up around my neck. "See you tonight," he said.

"Okay, Dad." Both of my parents, I thought, were coping the best they could.

"You're sure you're all right, Hopie?"

"I'm sure," I said. His voice was coming from somewhere near the door, but in the dark I couldn't tell if it was him I was talking to or his shadow. "I love you, Dad," I said, to the place where he seemed to be.

"Love you too, Hopie." My father turned and walked out the door, his long shadow trailing after him.

Six days later, when the stitches beneath my eyes were out and my mouth and cheeks had deflated to a more normal size, I secured a room in an apartment through a friend of a friend who was moving out of it.

I took only one medium-sized suitcase with me when I left. It surprised me that everything I wanted from my parents' home fit into such a limited space.

CHAPTER 9

D r. S— keeps the glossy black-and-white headshots of his clients pinned to a bulletin board in his office. The faces, mostly young women, smile out at him like individual radiant suns. Some are familiar; most are not. He likes to pause in front of the board, his arm around me as we come out of the exam room, and talk about his more famous patients.

"Here's someone you'll know," he says, jabbing a finger at a pretty, garden-variety blonde in a bikini. "The new *Baywatch* girl. I just did her breasts."

I know, from my grandfather, that it isn't ethical for a doctor to name his patients. Still, each of the photographs has been inscribed by its owner with a glib, private remark like "Dear Bob, Shut Up!!! Love, Valerie." The sheer quantity of the photographs astonishes me, not because I am surprised at the number of wannabe actors and models in Los Angeles, but because apparently, Dr. S— does not take down any of the pictures, just pins the newer ones on top of the old like some sort of collage. Tacked atop one another, the perfect faces resemble the pattern of a pretty wallpaper which has not been very well matched at its seams. After a few minutes of staring at the board, their flawlessness becomes less compelling than simply generic, manufactured. The French have a term for a woman who is unconventionally beautiful: *belle laide.* Beautiful ugly. None of the faces on Dr. S—'s bulletin board are *belle laide,* just *belle.* Each face projects, along with its appeal, a carefully calculated attitude: *approachable, sexy, wholesome, exotic.* I wonder how many roles of film clicked by, how many poses had to be affected in order to achieve the perfect degree of nuance.

At the bottom perimeter of the bulletin board I notice a couple of snapshots, tacked carelessly. They look amateurish and inconsequential beside the glossy professional ones. Peering closer, I see that one of the photographs is of a middle-aged, moderately attractive woman and two small, dark-haired girls, both of whom have Dr. S—'s smile.

"Is that your—?" Dr. S— does not wear a wedding ring. "Your family?"

"My ex-wife, Jeanette. And those are my girls."

"They're cute," I say. "What are they, three and five?"

"Something like that. Little devils, is what they are." Dr. S— chuckles, and I wonder if he really does not know the ages of his children. He looks at me. "We're still very close, my wife and I."

Does he notice he's dropped the "ex"—affectionately, or out of habit?

"She's an interior designer. Her business is booming, and she's never looked better."

"That's great," I say, wondering why I should be happy for his ex-wife.

"I have that effect on women. Always have." Dr. S— shrugs affably, as if bewildered by his own Pygmalion-esque powers. "Every woman I've ever known has improved herself in some way from knowing me. And I don't mean just physically, as you might imagine! My fiancée got a big promotion just weeks after we met."

"Fiancée?" The word feels like a cannonball slug to my gut, a reaction which surprises me with its intensity.

"Margo. Haven't you met her? She's always dropping by here."

"No." It takes me a moment to recover. It's much more painful to imagine the immediacy of Dr. S—'s fiancée, whatever she may look like, than the two-dimensional paper-doll perfection of the women on the bulletin board. "What does she—I mean, Margo—do?"

"She's a vice president of marketing at Dress Barn."

"Ah." What, not an actress or model? This surprises me, but it gives me hope, too. If Dr. S— can fall in love with someone not famous, not glamorous, someone who works for a chain of discount stores, then why not with me?

My eyes settle on the snapshots of Dr. S—'s ex-wife and children. In one picture, slightly out of focus, the boys have their arms wrapped around the bristly neck of a large animal.

"Is that a . . . horse?" I ask.

"A donkey. Eddie. I lost him in the divorce." Dr. S— sounds rueful. "He's a miniature donkey. Best pet you could ever have. Clean, friendly, no trouble at all."

It occurs to me that Dr. S— could, in fact, be describing his ideal woman.

"Isn't it ironic," he says, "that a man like me who makes people beautiful for a living would choose an ass for a pet?"

I am capable of telling myself many lies, but I am not enough of a fool to believe that Dr. S— is Prince Charming. The spell he weaves is of equal parts attraction and revulsion. My attraction to him oddly seems to increase in direct proportion to my disgust. Why? Perhaps these opposing emotions, forced into such close proximity in the brain, create an alchemy that bewitches. Is this odd chemical mix the secret to Dr. S—'s magnetism? Certainly, it is not his skill as a surgeon that accounts for his popularity. There are many more skilled, far more qualified plastic surgeons in Los Angeles. What is it about Bob S—?

Dr. S— is, as he himself likes to say, an enigma. A Renaissance man. He is so many things. For instance, he writes songs. He has one which he is certain would be perfect for Celine Dion, if only he could get it to one of her handlers. I don't, by any chance, know anyone who knows someone who might know her, do I?

Dr. S— does not believe in the bonds of the traditional doctor-patient relationship. His clients are many things to him. They are his patients, of course, but they are also his audience, his fan club and, he is fond of saying, his friends. Dr. S— has an open-door policy. You do not need an appointment to stop by his office, though even if you do have one, you may not get more than two seconds of his time. You may have to wait a long time to see him, too, because Dr. S— likes to get in a game or two of tennis before work in the mornings and sometimes at lunch. He likes to keep his priorities straight. He insists on a healthy mix of business and pleasure. For this reason, Dr. S— does not mind keeping his patients waiting while he finishes a particularly challenging set. They will wait. It doesn't matter, either, if he has to push back a surgery by an hour or two or three. It is, after all, his surgical suite. Patients, nurses, anesthesiologist: They must all wait. Whether you work for Dr. S— or you want him to work on you, you will learn to wait. He considers his malleable business hours a plus for his patients. If, for example, the only time that you can have your breasts enlarged happens to be seven on a Friday night? Not a problem. Drop by at that hour and you'll smell the take-out Chinese food wafting through the O.R. If you ask nicely, Dr. S— might even let you watch as he performs surgery (though this privilege is usually reserved for his relatives, and friends of his relatives). He is, after all, an artist. Just don't spill your wonton soup on the surgical tray.

Lacking the confidence to just drop by breezily, I often construct some small excuse to show up at Dr. S—'s office. One morning, it is an article I read in a magazine about a woman in Europe who was having her face and body surgically resculpted to resemble the works of the great masters of art. Mona Lisa's perfect aquiline nose; Botticelli's apple cheeks; jutting breasts like those of the marble torso of Winged Victory. She was a sculptor, this woman, and though she would not be doing the actual sculpting herself in this case, her finished face and body would be her exhibit.

Though I waited nearly two hours that morning, I never considered leaving and coming back at a later time. Being in Dr. S—'s office is better than being alone in my apartment. It is better than being anywhere. His waiting room has become my haven. It resembles, I think, less a doctor's office than a bachelor's tasteful, slightly eclectic living room. The pale green walls lend an underwater, vaguely embryonic feel. The teal leather sectional sofa curves around a heavy teak coffee table, which is stacked high with magazines and several large arty books, one of which features black-and-white photographs of parts of a woman's body transposed against wonders of the natural world, like the curve of a hip against a sand dune. On a stand in one corner is a large, colorful papier-mâché puffer fish—a whimsical touch, I think, which shows his childish side.

I want to believe that Dr. S— spends even a fraction of the time thinking about me as I do about him, though I know this is unlikely. Nevertheless I can't help feeling that I deserve some degree of intimacy. How can I *not* feel a more than casual connection? I have, after all, made myself more vulnerable to this man than I have to any lover. He has seen me looking my absolute worst: bruised, bloody, without makeup, and still he said, *You look great! Look at you!* He has bent over my supine body like the prince over Snow White. He has used all his skill and attention to make me into something more desirable than what I am. He has both inflicted and taken away pain. Doesn't such intimate contact merit a special, even sacred, sort of bond? What more vivid demonstration of love is there, after all, than suffering willingly at the hands of another?

Sitting in Dr. S—'s office, I realize the extent of my infatuation. I hope, with every cell of my body, that he and I can one day be more than doctor and patient. That there will be an *us.* Doesn't all my time and effort merit *something* other than the sterile doctor-patient relationship? Didn't Bob S— himself say to me, *Our relationship does not end when you leave my operating room?*

Even after two and a half hours of waiting, my hope does not waiver, though my patience does. The *Vogue* magazine in my lap, barely glanced at, is open to an article titled "The New Black Is . . . Black!" The teenage model wears a short black dress; her legs are so thin they resemble a wishbone. Every now and then I look up at the frosted glass partition, etched with arching koi carp, which separates the waiting area from the receptionist's desk. From behind the glass comes the brisk sawing of a nail file. Occasionally, the phone rings, with the jarring shriek of a vase shattering.

Four other patients have been called in, two of whom arrived after I did. Twice I have watched Dr. S—'s silhouette appear behind the partition, my heart knocking hard in my chest as I wonder whether I am next. I watch him, a shadow figure behind the frosted glass, swing an arm over his head, slicing the air to show his receptionist how he serves a winning ace.

At eleven-thirty-three, his shadow appears again, and speaks. "When you have a chance, dear," he says, "would you mind ordering a cake from La Brea Bakery for Margo's birthday? We're going to the Ivy tonight, but I thought we'd do dessert at home."

Stunned, I think: *Margo? The fiancée? Is he planning to propose to her?*

Suddenly, I can't wait any longer to see him. Emboldened by desperation, I lunge for the receptionist's window, tap hard on the glass.

"Hope?" Dr. S— looks only mildly surprised to see me.

I thrust the article at him, my words tumbling out in a rush. "I thought you might like to read this."

"Great," he says. "Thanks."

Without glancing at it, Dr. S— thrusts the article toward his receptionist, who is too busy ordering the cake to notice. I watch as it floats, facedown, onto the floor by her desk.

"I'm running late," he says to me. "Are we seeing you today? Do you have an appointment?"

Stung, I feel my shoulders scrunch up to my neck. "No," I murmur. "I don't. I just wanted to . . ." But Dr. S— is no longer listening. He is looking over the receptionist's shoulder at his busy schedule, resting a hand on her arm.

I slink out the door into the hall, push the button for the elevator. *I hate you,* I think, looking at Dr. S—'s name on his door. *I hate you so much it feels like love, the same intensity.*

Alone in the elevator, tears rise in my eyes. My face, reflected in the steel walls, stretches and distorts as in a funhouse mirror.

I hate you. I mouth the words silently to my reflection. *Hate you hate you hate you.*

By the time the doors open at the underground garage, I am no longer talking to him, but to myself.

In my car I cry behind my sunglasses as I pay the parking attendant. All the way down Wilshire, to Sixth Street, I cry huge, unladylike sobs which frighten me with their force, racking my body, making driving difficult. I'm turning onto Irving Boulevard before I realize that I've headed home to my parents' house. Driving by, I see my mother's Mercedes in the driveway. The personalized plate on her car reads: 4VLUVC.

I could go in, I think. *I could go inside and confess everything and throw myself on her mercy. I could let her fold me under her wing and tell me what I've done wrong* (everything) *and what to do* (be charming, be beautiful, make her proud) *and who to be: her dazzling daughter in public, her sickly wounded bird in private.*

I keep going, like a stranger, like someone terribly lost, late, and in need of directions.

CHAPTER 10

Hugh Bishop wore a plaid bow tie that lit up from within and played a tinny version of "Joy to the World" when you pressed the knot. When I was growing up, holiday dinners were just about the only times we saw the Bishops at family, gatherings that were invariably stiff, awkward, and unpleasant for all involved.

Just as chickens and other fowl establish a pecking order which is unchanging and determines everything about the way each chicken relates to the others, so my father's extended family, too, had a certain established order. Each of us had a title and a role. My mother was the rogue. My grandmother was the genteel gentlewoman. My father was the good-natured goof. Amanda, the elder Bishop girl was musical, and Anna Bishop was simply the baby, eating olives off her fingers. I was the pretty one; Hugh's wife Helen had even called me that once, letting it slip out, I thought, in a tone that was more degrading than flattering. Helen herself was bossy and terrifying. Hugh was Professor Bishop, and my grandfather was God. I imagined each of us obediently folding ourselves into our individual containers, from which we would spring like jack-in-the-boxes in each others' presence. I wondered if any of them felt as miserably locked into their roles as I did, though I supposed it made life easier for everyone by taking some of the guesswork out of the way we related to one another. Our pecking order made relations between us, if not less strained, at least more predictable.

My mother's desire for me to be glamorous, stunning, and charming—to dazzle my father's family—added to the pressure I already heaped upon myself. It took an enormous amount of time and effort to make myself beautiful, about two and a half hours of preparation. I spent far more time on my appearance than I did on my schoolwork. I did moderately well with a minimum of effort at the private, all-girls high school I attended; a recent English class had reignited my interest in creative writing, and I often scribbled out thoughts or parts of stories in my journal. I also enjoyed French, which I had been studying since seventh grade in Hong Kong. Language came easily to me and I was in the Advanced Placement French class. But none of these interests seemed as compelling or urgent to me as being beautiful. I always kept it in the back of my mind that I would, someday, pursue writing, but I had much more immediate concerns.

Because there were no boys at my school, and because a universally unflattering uniform was required, I engaged in only minimal preparations each morning. But for any event at which I might be seen by men, even a family gathering, my "beauty routine" took on a ritualistic complexity. It actually started the night before, when I would apply a coat of self-tanner to my face and entire body. Being tan, in Los Angeles, was an integral part of being attractive. My parents belonged to a beach club in Santa Monica, and I was always ashamed at my skin's inability to become anything other than a livid red. My discovery of self-tanning cream was akin to a miracle. I applied it every other night, a process which involved first showering and exfoliating every inch of my body, then drying off and applying the unpleasant-smelling lotion with painstaking care so that my skin would not betray me with any tell-tale streaks. Finally, I would have to stand around naked in my room for at least fifteen minutes while the lotion dried. Slipping between the sheets, I prayed I would not sweat.

The next morning, I regarded my tanned face in the mirror with infinite satisfaction. But this was only step one in my routine. Next, I took another shower, washing off as much of the self-tanning-cream-smell as I could. Then a facial moisturizer, and a scented moisturizer for the body. Wrapped in my robe, I focused on my makeup: curled eyelashes; concealer under the eyes (always pat the delicate skin gently, using your ring finger); a bit of foundation on other parts of the face; set the whole thing with powder; dust off excess powder to avoid the dreaded and aging masklike look; add a few strokes of blush; line and shadow the eyes; two coats (at least) of mascara; lip pencil to enlarge the border of my lips; lipstick. Finally, a soft swipe over my skin with a clean cotton ball to remove any excess makeup and assure that I had the obligatory (according to the magazines) "natural look." I performed this routine in exactly this sequence, without fail, never skipping a step or altering the order. If my concentration wavered, my confidence shattered.

After blow-drying my hair, the final step in my beauty routine, I would dress. I usually chose my clothes for their ability to show off my body, but I was far less concerned with what I wore than I was with my face. My face was like the sun, around which all other elements of my attractiveness revolved, secondary in importance and dependent. I did not like to be disturbed when performing any part of my routine, but especially not when I was concentrating on my makeup, a concentration close to meditation. A haphazardly applied coat of mascara could ruin *everything*, not just my appearance; if I lost focus, I would lose my mental momentum as well, the mysterious and incantation-like psyching-up I did along with my makeup. There wasn't anything specific I said to myself as I primped, but I was addicted to the feeling of increasing joy and confidence as I made myself beautiful. It was, in every way, an emotional as well as a physical process.

Perhaps because of the effort I put into it, I was convinced that my beauty was all smoke and mirrors, an illusion which might fail at any moment. I was not at all a natural beauty; a *real* beauty would spring from the bedsheets every morning as fresh and stunning as Aphrodite emerging from the sea on her clamshell. My attractiveness was an illusion, the product of lotions and pencils and compacts full of powder, not to mention the hours I spent at the hairdresser's each month having my long hair streaked white-blonde. My own insecurities, combined with my mother's desire for me to dazzle, made time spent with my father's family feel like a test of my abilities as a magician.

Part of my role, or perhaps proof that I had succeeded in my role, was enduring Hugh's unwelcome attention. Every Thanksgiving, Christmas, and Easter, Hugh's eyes poured over me like the sticky glaze on the ham, clinging to my breasts and legs. He always rushed to help me off with my coat, standing so close behind me his warm breath puffed on my neck, his hands sliding down my arms as he slid the coat off my shoulders. Seated across the dinner table from him, there was no escape from his smirking eyes, which made me feel as if I had gravy smeared on my mouth. It disturbed me to know that he was a professor of law at a major university, a man who stood in front of his students every day explaining right from wrong. My skin crawled under what I imagined to be the explicitness of his thoughts.

Worse, even, than holiday dinners was the occasional summer pool party at the Bishops' Hancock Park home. My mother encouraged me to wear string bikinis, to show off my "cute shape"; in the swimwear section of Bullock's Wilshire, she pulled the skimpiest suits from the racks. Any trepidation I expressed at the thought of appearing in public with so little to cover me my mother brushed away with clucking *tsk-tsk*s: "Don't you know how *lucky* you are to have such a great figure? Most models would *kill* for a body like yours!" I willingly went along with her suggestions, realizing that part of her enthusiasm had to do with the fact that the Bishop girls were still pudgy in their Speedos. It was only when I emerged from the Bishops' pool that I doubted my mother's choice. Three tiny triangles of fabric were not enough to hide me from Hugh's stare. There was only so long I could avoid Hugh's stare by lingering in the pool, safely hidden underwater with the sun beating down on my shoulders, before my body turned into a waterlogged plum. As I dashed for a towel I caught my reflection in the twin mirrored lenses of Hugh's sunglasses. He looked like Erik Estrada from CHiPs, smarmy and leering. My mother said Hugh's vanity was so great that he slept in a hair net—How did she know this?—and used a sun lamp to stay tan. His wife Helen and their two daughters called him Professor Bishop instead of Dad, a source of hilarity to my mother, who parroted their chirpy voices all the way home. My mother said that Hugh had once tried to "play footsie" with her, years ago, when she first met him. She had laughed it off. This was not something I wanted to have in common with my mother, both of us having been the recipient of Hugh's unwanted advances. But I knew my mother would see it this way, another bond between us, another solidarity in the face of the Hathaways.

But if my parents noticed Hugh's untoward attentions—how could they not?—they didn't mention it. I dropped hints about Hugh's perversion but it was impossible to crack the surface of my mother's mockery. They joked that, yes, Hugh was probably "checking me out," but could you blame him? "He's probably never *seen* such a gorgeous thing," my mother cackled. "He just can't *help* himself." A gorgeous *thing*? I was a pretty knick-knack, to be picked up, palmed casually, and put back. It was funny; why couldn't I laugh?

Unchecked, Hugh's attention toward me spread like a stain. His hand crept across the tablecloth to brush mine every time he reached for the butter. He became bolder about leaning in to make private, innuendo-laced comments when he removed my coat. "Allow *me*," and "*May* I, Hopie?" became, when uttered into my neck with his hushed, hot-breathed, not-so-subtle suggestions. The Christmas when I was sixteen, we went on our first and only vacation with my father's family and the Bishops to the Awahnee Hotel in Yosemite. My parents and I spent Christmas day cross-country skiing. My cheeks stung from snow and sun and the attention of a boy I'd met. In the middle of the third course of the Bracebridge Dinner, the boy came over to our table to talk to me. We agreed to meet after dinner for a soda, the teenager's version of a nightcap. Our table fell into an eager hush as we made our plans. It irked me that the Hathaways and the Bishops did not bother to conceal their interest in my social life, as if it were a suitable entertainment for them.

When the boy left to go back to his table, there was an expectant silence. Feeling the flush of my sun-burned cheeks grow deeper, I turned my eyes to the faraway beams of the room's vaulted ceiling.

"Is that Hope's latest heartthrob?" Helen's voice was shrill and as subtle as a foghorn.

I was embarrassed, but I did not expect my mother to defend me, because she was openly boastful about how many dates I went on. I had been allowed to date at fifteen and had not stopped since. The main criteria for who I went out with was that they asked me. Yet in spite of all this, my physical experience with boys consisted only of kissing and what my health teacher had called "light petting." I resolutely refused to go further, entertaining the idea that I would have to be madly in love in order for a boy to be "the one." I was aware of the disparity between what I actually had done, sexually, and what the Bishops must have imagined I had. It made me uneasy, but it was not something I could discuss with my mother. Sexuality, mine in particular, was oddly off-limits for her. I had once asked her, as casually as I could, what she would think of me going on the pill. My two best girlfriends had gone on it at sixteen, one of them with the full support of her mother. My mother said to me, "You can do whatever it is you want to do, but I do not want to know about it." End of conversation.

When Helen asked about "my heartthrob," laughter rippled around our table. In spite of her reticence to discuss all things sexual with me, my mother always found a way to make mention, especially to my father's family, of my many dates, creating a scandalous image of myself, which I was uncomfortable with. Wrapped up in her own insecurity, I think she wanted me to be a sort of grenade thrown amongst the staid Hathaways and Bishops, attracting the attention she herself felt denied or unworthy of. But this put me in a difficult position. I understood, even then, that a pretty young flirt is often construed as sexually promiscuous whether or not she is, and that thinking of me this way may have made me seem less threatening to Helen and her girls. Perhaps it was for this reason, as a kind of unconscious protest against the way in which I was perceived, that I held on to my virginity with a stubborn pride until my first year of college, long after my girlfriends had lost theirs. I knew how the Bishops saw me and I knew, too, that I helped perpetuate their opinion. I *was* a flirt, seeking out male attention like a heat-seeking missile. I wore teeny bikinis. I dated constantly. Even though I was not at all the sort of girl they envisioned, I still nurtured a secret shame within myself. Labels like *slut, easy,* and *tease* floated around accusingly in my head.

My mother had once made an odd confession to me, saying that she had "a reputation" in high school. "I worked my way through the whole baseball team," she said, with a mixture of shame and pride. Her mother, my grandmother, made a similar boast: She had collected the pins of five fraternity boys. It was odd, these thinly veiled admissions of promiscuity from two women who paid such bold lip service to female independence, often ridiculing the ineffectualness of their husbands and men in general. Their actions betrayed a cloying neediness. The message was confusingly twofold: *Men are trophies. Sling another notch on your belt and move on.* And: *You must have a man at all times. You are not a complete person without one. Cast your line out for a suitable candidate and reel him in!*

That night at the Awahnee, Hugh rose from his chair, saying he had to go to "the little boys' room." Dread crept along my spine. Earlier in the day, I had been summoned to Helen and Hugh's room on some contrived errand; when Hugh answered the door, he was wearing only a towel around his waist, a cowboy hat, and a leer. Now, as he passed my chair, he leaned down close, his fruity gin-laced breath misting my ear.

"*Hard* throb," he whispered.

Later that night, in my parents' room, I told them about Hugh's comment, the words spilling out in a rush.

"Gross," my mother said. "Clayton! Come in here."

My father appeared in the bathroom doorway, brushing his teeth. There are few men who dress thoroughly and formally for bed, and my father is one of them—maroon silk bathrobe with monogrammed pocket, pin-striped Brooks Brothers pajamas, socks, and slippers.

My mother began to giggle. "Listen to what Hugh said to your daughter."

My father brushed vigorously as my mother told the story, the toothpaste foaming into a huge, clownish white outline around his mouth. When she finished, he went into the bathroom and spit loudly into the sink. "Swell guy," he called out. He gargled, then spit again.

The bubble of anger that had been swelling steadily in my chest since dinner burst.

"Jesus, Dad!" I cried. "Don't you *care* about this? Do you think it's *funny* that Hugh pervs on me?"

My mother was eyeing me as if it was, in fact, very funny, and my reaction was the funniest thing of all.

"Don't either of you give a shit that your friend keeps coming on to me?" I was near tears, but in spite of my anger my voice sounded whiny and indignant in my ears, a child's silly complaint.

"Ah, listen." My mother's eyes still sparkled, but she was in sympathy mode. She patted the spot next to her on the bed, but I refused to sit down. "C'mon, sweet apple. Don't you see how absurd this all is? The great Professor Bishop, drooling over his friend's teenaged daughter. What do you think the Hathaways' fancy friends would think about *that?*"

"I don't care a *fuck* about the Hathaways' fancy friends! I care that my mother and father, who are supposed to protect me— Hello? *Is anyone listening to me?*"

"Uh-huh." My mother's attention was on the television, where the jaunty intro to *Masterpiece Theatre* blared out. My father had retreated back into the bathroom, this time shutting the door.

I looked at my mother, bobbing her head to the music, and wanted to strangle her. She felt as distant from me as a satellite.

"I'm going to bed," I said. Defeat, despair, anger—the quickest escape route, I had learned, was sleep.

My mother cared more about humiliating the Hathaways than about my feelings; this stung more than a slap. Years later, I would read that holding a grudge is the grown-up version of throwing a temper tantrum. There was a story my mother told about her first meeting with the Hathaways, a tale elevated by her to the realm of legend like so many others, spun and polished into myth. The first time she arrived to meet them, my mother was wearing a baby-blue boiled-wool suit with matching pillbox hat and white gloves with pearl buttons at the wrists, an ensemble purchased especially for the trip. Standing on my grandparents' doorstep, fresh out of the first taxi ride she had ever taken, my mother extended her gloved hand to my grandmother. As she did, the little hat tumbled off her head and landed on the ground, next to one of my grandmother's shoes.

Lying there upturned, my mother said, "That hat looked just like a beggar's cup, fallen at the grand lady's feet." She found something symbolic in this. There must have been a moment when the two women stared at the hat; I picture it lying there like a rice bowl, rocking slightly back and forth. My grandmother stared at it, and my mother stared at it, and a tiny contest was born. After what I imagined must have been a very long minute, my mother bent down and picked it up. Carrying this newly minted symbol of her impoverishment in her hands, my mother strode stiffly across the threshold of the Hathaways' home. "I entered that goddamned house like some poor sucker asking for alms," she said.

I didn't know how much of this story was true and how much was my mother's exaggeration, and I don't think it mattered to her. When she told it, the story gave her eyes a glow that looked almost serene, like contentment.

A few months after the "hard throb" incident, we went to Easter dinner at the Bishops' house. I remember feeling relieved when the evening passed with only a few smirks from Hugh. When the meal was over, I got up to carry my plate to the kitchen. As I set it in the sink, I felt a presence behind me in the empty kitchen. I knew who it was without turning around. He came up behind me, so close that the prickly smell of his cologne caught in my nose, causing me to sneeze.

"God bless you, Hopie," he said.

Without another word, Hugh drew back my hand and put it on the front of his pants. His gesture shocked me into silence as surely as if he'd put his hand over my mouth.

His crotch felt lumpy, like a bag of pecans. I tried to wrench my hand free, but he held it there. A little sigh like a moan escaped his lips. I was surprised by the strength of his grip, that his small hand could be so strong.

"Professor Bishop!"

We turned, Hugh and I, to see Helen standing in the doorway. Her hands were on her hips. She wafted anger and her favorite perfume, Fracas.

"Professor Hugh Bishop," she said again, briskly, though her eyes were on me. "You are needed in the dining room to cut the raspberry tart."

Hugh scuttled quickly out of the kitchen, but Helen continued to stand there. Her face was livid; her blonde hair looked like it had been set in a Jell-O mold. Her simmering look said that although dessert was being served in the other room, the real tart was here in the kitchen.

"You," she said, her voice so calm and low I could barely hear her, "are going to get exactly what you deserve."

One of my knees was shaking. What was it I deserved? I half wanted her to tell me. I was ready to believe anything. My father said Helen had once called him a "mongoloid idiot." My mother always chastised my father for being intimidated by her, but I could see that same Helen now, cruel and terrifying.

She turned and swept out of the kitchen.

I leaned over the sink, reeling with fear, shame, and a sort of dread. Helen's words spun around in my head like a gypsy's mysterious curse. What was it I deserved?

Beside me on the counter was a bottle of scotch, open and half full. Without thinking I turned it up to my lips, closing my eyes against the honey-colored burn. Through the kitchen window, across the patio, I saw that a light rain had started. Helen's two dogs huddled together under the patio table. They were Welsh Corgies, Helen's pride and joy. She loved them as much as my grandmother loved her roses, boasting about their AKC papers and the purity of their bloodlines. My mother said that if Helen could have gotten her dogs into Stanford, she would have. Each one had a long, silly show name, Sir Lucky's Irish Pride this-and-that and Lady Melanie of Something-or-other. They were not, to me, particularly impressive dogs, in spite of Helen's boast that the Queen of England herself kept Corgies. As I watched, Sir Lucky climbed atop Lady Melanie and began humping away with a furious abandon that undermined his rarified pedigree. Lady Melanie, nonplussed, sniffed at a puddle on the concrete. Apparently, she understood something I didn't: Male sexual attention, however unwanted and inappropriate, was something to be endured, ignored, or dismissed with a shrug.

I leaned over and vomited into the sink.

Sunk into the backseat of my parents' car on the way home, still nauseous, I tried to turn what had happened into words. *Hugh pressed himself into me.* The words collected on my tongue, heavy and bitter as river stones. To my mother's ears they would be a burst of confetti, a boast. The words would come out all wrong, I was sure, twisted and confused—my fault.

My mother slept and my father drove faster than usual, his car gliding smoothly over the black, rain-soaked streets. After a while I stopped thinking. I found that if I narrowed and unfocused my eyes, the world became a blur of lights outside my window, and I didn't feel so sick.

CHAPTER 11

"Are you sure the directions say to turn *left* on Ocean View?" my roommate Anita asks, pulling her car onto the shoulder of Mulholland Drive.

"Straight up to the top of Outpost, left on Mulholland, right on Ocean View," I read. "First left on Pacific Trail, and the house should be right there."

Anita swings back onto Mulholland, accidentally cutting off a black BMW that comes speeding around a curve, blaring its horn at us.

"Jerks." Anita swipes her hand across her forehead as the car races past us. "Between the heat and these drivers, this is a nightmare."

We are on our way to a party in the Hollywood Hills. It is a sticky, freakishly hot winter night. For days the clouds overhead have promised, but not delivered, the relief of rain.

"Here! This should be it." Anita pulls up in front of an enormous white stucco monstrosity covered in bougainvillea. The house is built into the jagged hillside in tiers, balanced atop wooden stilts. In the dusk, the spindly looking pillars look like straws.

"Wow," Anita says. "I wouldn't want to be under there when the Big One hits."

The hot weather is making everyone think of earthquakes; even the scientists are making predictions. My roommates and I live in fear of the inevitable Big One that will slide us all the way to Malibu.

We find a parking spot down the narrow street and have to hike uphill, squeezing ourselves flat against parked cars every time another car drives by.

"Do you know anyone who's going to be here?" I ask her, starting to feel panicky.

"Possibly. A guy in my Child Development class said he might show up."

I want to ask Anita whether she would mind if I held her hand when she stops me, her hands on my shoulders.

"Wait! Makeup check." Anita studies my face. "You look fine," she says. "But I'm melting." She licks a finger and runs it under each eye, checking for mascara smears.

Of the three roommates, Anita is the only one with whom I've formed a friendship. She is at home almost as much as I am, so there is really no way for us to avoid each other. More than sheer proximity, though, is the fact that we share a vagueness, an uncertainty, an insecurity which is as alike as our backgrounds are different.

In a heart-shaped frame on her dresser, Anita keeps a picture of herself accepting an award from her hometown farming club back in Minnesota. A little scrolly script at the bottom of the picture reads: 4-H Dairy Princess. Anita believes that anything is possible with a resolute attitude and a full face of Covergirl makeup. She is studying Early Childhood Education at UCLA, taking just a couple of classes at a time and using the rest of the money her father sends her for tuition to indulge her passion for makeup, CDs, and food. She says, though I do not believe her and I sense she does not really believe herself, that what she really wants to be is an actress. She is certain that she will be discovered while walking down the street one day, just like in the stories of old Hollywood. "As soon as I lose weight," she says. "Just as soon as I lose weight." The poignancy in her words draws me closer to her. Both of us are waiting for our lives to begin as soon as a big If Only comes true. Our If Only's are as big and shapeless as clouds, but they both involve being *seen*, being *discovered*. We insist that they are the reason why we keep happiness at arm's length. I wonder, sometimes, whether if each of us were offered what it is we claim to want so desperately, would we have the courage to take it? And would it even satisfy? Would Anita be happy as a skinny starlet, and would I be content if I were flawlessly beautiful? I have learned this: Wanting fills up the emptiness inside you as much or even more than actually having something. Wanting is hope. Having is disappointment.

Walking up to the party, I think about what an odd pair we make, like a bad joke. *Did you hear the one about the Deb and the Dairy Princess?* I can feel Anita's nervousness, and I want to tell her she is beautiful, but I know she won't believe me. I really think that Anita *is* beautiful in her zaftig way, which makes her as different from the scrawny Los Angeles women as an orchid from a palm tree. I am always easier on other women's looks than I am on my own, more willing to appreciate the unconventional, or to forgive a flaw. But my generosity does not apply to myself.

Up close, the party house is so thoroughly covered in climbing bougainvillea that it appears as if it is being devoured by purple blossoms. The smell of pot and clove cigarettes carries out to us on the heat-heavy air. Inside, Anita and I reel for a moment, adjusting to the thump of music and crush of people. Looking around at the guests, I think: Assorted Beautiful People. Actor and model types. A few glance in our direction, but for the most part everyone wears looks of such studied vacuity, one wonders whether they even have a pulse. A grenade could go off and still they wouldn't react. It has

always struck me as odd that among the wanna-be actors and actresses in Los Angeles, emotion of any kind is so decidedly uncool.
Shouldn't people whose livelihood depends upon believably emot-
ing strong feelings at least demonstrate a few of their own? Or does
enthusiasm of any kind make you too vulnerable? I could never
master that attitude of surly boredom; I am too much the
wholesome girl next door, too ready to smile, too eager to please. I
look at the party guests with their expressions of haughty detachment, holding their cigarettes and their angular bodies like props,
and feel a mix of fear and envy. Why can't I be like them? Why
can't I at least *act* as if I don't give a shit what other people think of
me? As it is, I often feel like an eager puppy dog, panting after
everyone's approval. Emotion is something I give away too easily. I
need everyone's approval so badly that every encounter, however
brief and inconsequential, feels like a performance. Charming a
surly store clerk is an acid test of my worth. The effort this takes is
exhausting, yet only lately has it struck me how scattered I feel. It
feels as if I am handing out little parts of myself, bits and pieces I
can never get back. I've become a handful of loose change jangling
around in my pocket. I am choking on my compulsive need to
please everyone, but it is a sickness, this need for applause. A scowl,
an indifferent glance can blow me to bits. With each encounter I
become smaller, more splintered, as I am leaving fragments of myself all over the city. Inside I'm quaking with anxiety; outside I'm
the picture of sunny loveliness. Who is this cheery stranger? Often,
I have to crawl under the covers of my bed and will myself back together. I feel like that villain in one of the *Terminator* movies—he
is shot to smithereens by Arnold, his body scattered into bits of
molten metal, but after a few minutes all the little blobs coalesce
and he is whole again. I feel compelled to vomit out a sunny effer-
vescence to everyone I meet, operating, as I do, under the assump-
tion that each person automatically does not like me, and it is up to
me to change their mind. I have become so lost in this dance to
please, I don't know what it is I really feel in any situation. As I

look around at the cool, aloof party guests, I think, *Why can't I keep whatever it is I feel, my essence, inside of me, to be taken out only for those I want to show it to, instead of turning myself inside out for every stranger's approval? Do I even know what my essence is? What is it I really feel?*

Anita immediately drifts away from me, having spotted someone she knows. I barricade myself in a corner of the dining room between the buffet table and a wall. My customary anxiety is tempered by the nauseousness I felt in Anita's hot car, and I am grateful to be distracted from all-out panic by a feeling that I might throw up. My anxiety always starts the same way, with a jolt of self-consciousness, as I realize that I am visible to the rest of the world. I freeze, my legs stiffen, my movements become jerky and robotic. I feel like one of those fainting goats, who stiffen and fall over when frightened. I fear I may faint, or in some way lose control of my mind and body. My vision wavers; lights are too bright. I want to hide. I feel myself starting to reel, and want to grab at something, or hide in a small space. Worse, even, than the panic itself is the thought that everyone might see my loss of control, my sheer helplessness.

With the way I feel, it's a wonder that I ever go out, let alone to a party. But one of the hallmarks of my anxiety is its unpredictability; there are days when I breeze through the grocery store with only a few twinges of fear; other times, I feel fine leaving the house but am blindsided as soon as I encounter another person. Perhaps I have more control over my phobias than I'm willing to admit, because the bottom line is this: When I really want to do something, I do it, anxiety or not. As in the case of tonight's party, sheer boredom has drawn me out of the apartment.

Perhaps because it helps to assuage my feeling of isolation, I am fascinated by stories of all manner of phobics, and the theories behind their mania, the more bizarre the better. They reassure me I am not alone in my craziness. I am particularly amused by the fact that doctors in the Victorian era believed that a woman's "hysteria" was caused by a wandering uterus. Who came up with that absurd image, a jaunty pear-shaped uterus lugging itself around the body, the twin ovaries like small suitcases in tow? *Only a man, I think, only a man could misunderstand a woman enough to come up with something like that.*

I am not hungry—panic always suppresses my appetite—but to look like I have a reason for haunting the buffet table, I pluck a tortilla chip from the vast array of food, so perfect and untouched it looks like set dressing in a movie: pink slabs of sushi, prawns speared with toothpicks, a pyramid of vermilion strawberries. Strawberries in the middle of winter? Here in Los Angeles, we are the recipients of a ridiculous bounty. Across the table, I notice a man staring at me. He is not staring so much as looking at me shyly, in glances. He is very tall, wearing a tight black T-shirt and jeans, and muscular in that self-conscious weight-lifter's way, as if every muscle has been sculpted for maximum impact. His furtive look is at odds with his bulky macho-man physique. He has the standard-issue Malibu Ken tan and an artfully moussed swell of blond hair. I guess him to be about thirty-five.

"Hiya." With a few long strides, he comes around the buffet table to me. "I'm Hank."

Like my mother, when I am feeling nervous, a tiny, critical, belittling voice asserts itself in my head. I think: *Hank?* The name of someone who might be handy with small repairs around the house. "I'm Hope," I say.

"That's pretty. Is that really your name?"

I realize he means is this the name I was born with, or one I'd appropriated: a stage name. "It's my name," I say. "I'm not an actress or anything." *Only in Hollywood,* I think.

"You don't hear it too often. Isn't there a character called Hope on *Days*—"

"—*Of Our Lives.* Yep. Hope Brady." I don't tell him that his name makes me think of a plumber.

"Can I get you a drink, Hope?"

"Yes. Why, thank you." Suddenly, I've become Scarlett O'Hara.

He returns with a glass of Chardonnay and a couple of fat naked prawns curled in a cocktail napkin. When the prawn goes into my mouth, Hank's eyes zoom in for a close-up. At his suggestion, we wander out onto one of the home's decks, overlooking the San Fernando Valley. Hank leans against a railing; behind him, red Christmas lights blink on and off, on and off, like an endorsement. Perched over the Valley, the house ought to have a spectacular view; tonight, however, only a few lights wink, feebly and far away, through the grimy haze.

"Beautiful." Hank spreads out his arms toward the muted vista, making me wonder whether he had even glanced at it. "How would you like to look at this every night?"

"Would you mind if we went inside?" The deck feels as if it is wobbling unsteadily beneath my feet. How can anyone relax in a house like this, I wonder, knowing that underneath, a few shaky wooden pillars are all that separate you from the jagged earth?

Inside, we have to shout to be heard over the throbbing music. "Are you a model, Hank?" I know this will flatter him, though I suspect he isn't. He's a bit long in the tooth for modeling.

"Close," he shouts, predictably pleased. "I'm an actor."

He rattles off the names of a few movies he's been in, while I nod as if they ring a bell.

"All minor roles, but my agent says I'm going to be a leading man. It's just a question of the right part."

Ping. The hollow ring in his voice, the desperate edge; these I recognize. It is the same note I hear in my own voice, when I tell people I am "temporarily unemployed" or "just waiting for the right opportunity to come along." I feel something like a rush of warmth toward Hank.

"I'm sure you'll make it," I say, trying to sound sincere. I look down at the blushing prawn, pink and exposed in its napkin.

When Hank asks me what I do, I tell him this: I've just graduated and am looking for a job in journalism, or maybe public relations, or at least something in which I can combine my love of writing with my degree in communications. I am both pleased and startled by how convincing I sound.

Hank nods, watching my lips. His grin is lopsided. "So you're home a lot. Anyone special in your life?"

"No." I try to sound wistful, like this is a temporary and unaccustomed state. "I mean, I've got some roommates, but . . ." Hank, abruptly less timid, has started nibbling my ear. It tickles. "I thought you were shy," I say, pulling away.

"I'm not shy," he says, hot breath in my ear. "If you're not."

I want, then and there, to walk away from Hank, because I don't like him, I am not at all attracted to him, and because I sense something vaguely threatening and unsavory about him. But I don't. I am not assertive enough, true, but there is more: Just as I do in the plastic surgeons' offices, I immediately dismiss my misgivings as untrustworthy and unsubstantiated. I have become as adept at shutting down my intuition as an anorexic is at ignoring her hunger. In fact, I so thoroughly distrust my inner voice that often, I do the opposite of what it is telling me. I despise my inability to make decisions. Knowing myself to be weak and ineffectual, I seek out people whose desires are so large and powerful that they easily eclipse my own.

Before I know it, I've finished a third glass of Chardonnay. The wine, the prawns, and the smoke are making me woozy.

"I can tell you'd be wonderful in bed." Hank leans in close. "Because you're so comfortable with yourself."

This isn't what I expected. I want to slap him, but instead I think, *Don't be a prude; this is just a risqué compliment.* Laughing in a way I hope is reckless, I pull away. "Wouldn't you like to know." I say.

"I would *love* to know."

His breath is damp on my already humid neck. I think of Hugh Bishop saying, *Hard throb.* Instead of the old shiver of revulsion, though, I surprise myself by giggling.

Hank says, "You are so hot, baby."

Hank's lines have all the heat of a cheesy B-movie, I think. But I'm acting, too, remember? Protesting as gently as Marvell's coy mistress, I push him away.

After the fourth Chardonnay, Hank's advances become like swatting away a fly. When I protest, Hank withdraws his hand from my breast and his tongue from my mouth, seeming humbled and apologetic, and we converse for a few moments like normal people, discussing some neutral subject: current events, celebrities. Then, abruptly, Hank is at it again, fondling, grabbing. Clearly sex is where Hank's mind veers back to, no matter what, like an erotic homing device. Drunk, I'm able to think about this in the most remote and scientific of ways, like someone studying the mating habits of tropical fish. Hank reminds me of the dauntless, sex-crazed male guppies in my childhood fish tank, shimmying their bright tails in front of the females all day, being rebuffed, and shimmying again.

I look around for Anita, not really caring where she is. "I suppose I should find my . . ." I can't remember what I was going to say.

Hank's hand is massaging slow circles on my butt. "Does that feel good?"

It doesn't, really. It doesn't feel good or bad. It could be someone else's butt he's touching. Still, a noise like *Mmm* comes out of my lips. I want to tell him that I have no physical reaction to him whatsoever, and that I am not fully sure whether it is because I am pickled in alcohol or simply because I have no idea what I feel in any situation anymore. But it doesn't seem worth the trouble of trying to explain it, even to myself.

"Did you know," I say to him, suddenly full of drunken inspiration, "that my grandmother used to give me cranberry juice with a splash of vodka in it when I was eleven years old?"

Hank groans into my ear.

"I used to drink it sitting by my grandfather's koi pond, with my legs dangling in the cold water." Why am I telling him this? I have no idea, though it suddenly seems important. "My grand-mother said it was good to get children used to drinking when they were young. She said it was what the Italians did. Which is funny, since we aren't Italian."

There was something else my grandmother used to say to me about drinking; what was it? Ah, yes: "Three vodka and cranberry's and I just *sail* through dinner with your grandfather!" What did it take, I wonder, for her to sail through sex?

"Do you want another drink?" Hank asks.

I shake my head. "What time is it? I think I ought to find my roommate."

"I'll help you find her. I saw you two come in together. Cute, fat girl, right?"

"Anita's not fat," I say, hurt by his easy dismissal of her. "She's—" But Hank has charged ahead, not listening.

The swell of people coming up the stairs makes me press my back against the wall as we descend the stairs to the first floor. Hank keeps his hand on my wrist, and as we reach the landing he abruptly yanks me backward, into a small, dark room. The door closes and there is only a tiny sliver of light at our feet.

"Hank?" I cannot see my hand in front of my face; panic cuts through the buzz of alcohol. "Hank, what are you doing?"

"Relax." His voice is very close in the darkness. "I've been want-ing to get you alone all night."

As he presses me backward I realize we are in a coat closet; I hear the squeak of hangers, and am overcome with the smells of leather, briny sweat, perfume. Hank's fingers jab under my T-shirt. "Let me out right now," I say. "I feel really sick. I'm serious." Will vomiting on Hank deter him?

He pushes open the door, and light floods my eyes. "See?" he says gallantly. "You've got nothing to worry about with me." Press-ing the small of my back with his hand, he returns me to the noise and activity.

Anita retrieves me, then, and it is time to leave the party. When

Hank asks for my number, as I knew he would, I realize that I could give him a fake one, or simply refuse. I don't ever have to see him again, so what does it matter how he reacts?

"Here's a pen."

Is it indifference, or fatigue, or just knee-jerk gratitude that makes me scribble the seven digits on the cocktail napkin Hank holds out for me? I don't know, and my throbbing head is reason enough not to think too much about it. On the way home, while Anita drives and I pretend to sleep, I search for a more compelling explanation for my acquiescence. I think: I don't *like* Hank, but I don't *dis*like him enough to refuse. In the months to come, I will continue to question the dull, heifer-like passivity that overcomes me when I am around him. It's a state almost like anesthesia; I experience neither pleasure nor pain.

Much later, I will come to realize that it is not simply my indifference to Hank which makes me as malleable as clay, but something darker, more desperate and dangerous: Fearing that I am unlovable, I must settle, and be grateful for, simply being desired.

CHAPTER 12

The society page of the *Los Angeles Times* had this to say about my debutante ball:

Stepping through a floral arch, eighteen radiant Las Madrinas Debutantes in long gowns and evening gloves heard their names announced at the annual Christmas Ball at the Beverly Hilton, attended by eight hundred.

Fathers in white tie escorted their daughters around the dance floor to applause, before the grand curtsy and the father-daughter waltz, which all had practiced for hours. Then escorts were invited to the floor, and ultimately stags (those without dates) had their twirl around the ballroom, which was decorated with eugenia topiaries, roses, and strings of tiny lights. All danced to the wee hours to P. Sterling's Orchestra.

Stepping out the door of the limousine at the Beverly Hilton hotel, I looked at the Mexican valet holding the door for me and imagined how silly and frivolous this whole event must seem to him, all these well-dressed wealthy people who had probably spent more on their daughters' dresses than he earned in two months. What a shock it was to see the ballroom, which had been empty and as cavernous as an airport hangar when we'd rehearsed, now full of people and tables, the great room pulsing with talk and clinking glasses and laughter and exploding flashbulbs. The stage upon which the debutantes were to be presented was rather small and in the rear of the room, and when my name was announced and it was my turn to walk out into the blindingly bright lights, I could not see beyond a few feet in front of me. I heard the rustling and shifting of bodies. I concentrated on the little bits of silver tape they had put on the stage to tell us where we needed to walk and stand. At a certain point near the front of the dance floor, we were to stop before the crowd at large and deliver the so-called grand curtsy. The hardest part was negotiating the small set of stairs from the stage to the dance floor. The lights were so glaring and my fright was so great that when I reached the predestined spot I could barely make out the faces of the Las Madrinas committee seated in the front row, a group of about twelve women who had themselves been Las Madrinas Debs and who now oversaw the event each year. One of them was Helen Bishop, and I shivered under the hot intensity of her gaze, avoiding her eyes.

Because the debutantes were called in alphabetical order according to their last names, I was one of the last to walk onto the stage. I watched the other girls before me, studying their fidgety gestures. Eight of them had gone to my high school, though none of us had been particularly close friends. Our affected ennui united us more than the fact that we had gone to school together. We shared the somewhat beleaguered attitude that this was something tiresome and silly. We were doing it for our parents, and our parents' parents, a small, dwindling sector of old Los Angeles who needed to believe that the world they had grown up in still existed, if even for a few hours.

As each girl took her turn out on the stage, I was reminded of the little figurine inside a jewelry box that twirls tremulously when you open the lid. Each of us had her own way of dealing with nerves. One of the girls, the heiress to a newspaper fortune, was so drunk she wobbled on her heels. Before the event she had enveloped me in an unexpected, sloppy embrace and I'd smelled the sweetly acrid waft of alcohol coming from her skin and her breath. Another of the girls was loudly fussing, boasting it seemed, over how to keep the room she'd rented upstairs for herself and her boyfriend a secret from her parents. "Not that they'll suspect," she was saying. "But just in case I'm going to say that—" Her name was called, and she floated out onto the stage.

Because my legs were trembling, the curtsy I gave fell far short of the deep, graceful ideal which we had all practiced, in which one's right knee was supposed to graze the floor. My curtsy was a quick nervous bob. I knew it was inferior, and I felt ashamed; it was certainly not the grand curtsy we were supposed to deliver. My mother, though, was delighted. She thought that my abbreviated curtsy was deliberate, a gesture of disdain for the whole event. She would refer to it, later, as "that half-assed curtsy," or "the 'up-yours' of curtsies."

After the curtsy, each girl was met at the edge of the dance floor by her escort. My escort was my first real boyfriend, Rick, whom I'd met some months previously at a fraternity party. Rick was very tall like my father, with the fair skin and hair of his Dutch parents. He was a fifth-year senior, still unsure of his major, and from the moment I met him he had focused all of his otherwise vague and indecisive interest on me. I liked Rick, I thought that perhaps I even loved him, but I felt smothered by his attention. Although he had decided immediately that I was "the one" for him, I had no such certainties about him. As a freshman, I wanted to have many more romantic adventures before settling down. Still, I was not assertive enough to break away from him. Instead, in passive-aggressive retaliation, I had begun to treat him badly. When he took me out to an expensive dinner at a restaurant atop the Bonaventure Hotel, I told him I'd always thought the Bonaventure was tacky. Rick cried, and I felt terrible about what I'd done, but I had discovered a mean streak in myself which I seemed to have no control over. I was treating Rick much the way my mother treated my father in their courtship, though I did not see this at the time.

At the appropriate time, the stags cut in on the escorts. My stag was Travis Shaw, whom I'd known since kindergarten. We twirled around, trying to make small talk, ignoring the little beads of sweat on each other's faces. Finally, the fathers were summoned to the floor for the father-daughter waltz.

My father's white gloves made his big hands look huge, like those of a clumsy mime. He spun me around the hotel ballroom in a stiff lilting waltz, beneath a ceiling of white lights meant to simulate a night sky strewn with stars, while my mother watched from somewhere out of sight, beyond the hot white lights. She had complained incessantly before the ball about how little she liked her own dress, a long column of light-blue plaid taffeta. When I finally saw her, at dinner, I noticed that she had nervously managed to tug loose some of the stitches on one of the dress's capped sleeves.

For many years my parents kept, in a prominent place, an eight-by-ten photograph from that night in a sterling frame. In the photo, I stand in my long dress, flanked on either side by my parents. I am holding my bouquet of white roses. My father is leaning slightly down toward me, a habit he adopts both to compensate for his height and to assure that the top of his head will not be cut off in photographs. My mother's smile is stiff and her eyes crinkle convincingly; she looks a little as if she has just been pinched. The three of us look happy. It is a near-perfect photograph.

CHAPTER 13

There are big thrills and there are little ones. Opening a brand-new beauty magazine, I feel the same hopeful, twitchy sense of anticipation I get in the waiting room of Dr. S—'s office. *Vogue, Glamour, Mademoiselle;* it doesn't matter. Hope wafts off the crisp, unread pages like those scented perfume ads. I await the arrival of the new crop of magazines each month like a dope-sick junkie anticipating a fix. Reading about all the new products will activate an adrenaline rush of desire in my veins. I will devour every word of each ad and article about this skin cream or that mascara or powder which is absolutely new and unlike any that's come before and think: *I must have it.* I suppose some people feel this way about Lionel trains, or stamps, or coins. As the calendar creeps past the mid-point of each month, I begin the countdown as to how long it might be until the new magazines appear on store shelves. Because I tend to panic in large stores, it gives me a potent incentive to do my grocery shopping. I force myself to get through the shopping by promising myself a magazine, the way a mother entices her youngster to behave by promising a candy bar at the check-out lane. A glossy treat awaits me, with its own version of a sugar rush. My mouth practically waters as my eyes skim the headlines. "Summer Hair 101: The Best Tricks and Tips." Or "Beauty Boot Camp: So-so to Stunning in Two Weeks!" New *Vogue* as antidepressant: It really works, though the half-life is far too short. For as long as I'm flipping through those glossy pages, I am transported.

I am ritualistic, even obsessive, about my magazines. Knowing the power and magic of a new magazine, it is of the utmost importance that I keep it all to myself until I have perused it to my heart's content. Once, one of my roommates asked if she could borrow my new *Allure*. Her request felt like a fist to my stomach. What could I say? *No, you can't touch it until I've read every single page. The magic will escape, scatter like fairies if someone else opens the pages first.* For this reason, I always pick a magazine that is several into the stack, so I can be sure it has not yet been touched. Furtively, because I know this is obsessive, I will tilt the cover so that it catches the supermarket light and reveals any evidence of having been opened: a tiny crease, a smear of fingerprints.

Once home, I hole up in my room with my treasure, lock the door, and begin. I must not be disturbed. I hoard the magazine in my room like a bulimic with a box of Twinkies, stuffing myself in solitude. I must gorge myself, consume every page in a single two- to four-hour sitting.

My heart starts to race with urgency at the first shiny advertisement. A lip gloss that actually *plumps up* your lips? How wonderful, like an answered prayer! How soon can I get to the store and buy this miracle product? One company, Philosophy, at least has the honesty to call its product Hope in a Jar. I admire its frankness, but I wouldn't buy it; there's something indelicate about putting one's desperation in boldface on a label. I prefer a more subtle advertising strategy, even if—especially if—it contains unpronounceable scientific words I do not understand, do not *want* to understand, for to understand them would be to unravel the mystery. It is easier to believe a company's overinflated promises when its product contains "revolutionary" ingredients which promise to be the very latest breakthrough, the cutting edge of beauty technology.

I rush through the magazine, folding pages, scribbling notes, making lists. Usually, I earmark the articles and come back to them later: homework. The articles are not as exciting, because they are longer and require concentration, but they are important to me because they justify all the rest of the beauty fluff. I am *learning something*. They are the four ounces of lean chicken breast that compensate for the fries and milk shake, almost making a balanced meal. I feel a slight pride after finishing each one. If there were a Trivial Pursuit of beauty, I would win hands-down. On the history of makeup, for example: The Maybelline company was founded by a boy who mixed up coal dust and petroleum jelly for his sister to darken her eyelashes with. How many people know *that?* Or this: The geishas used a deadly lead-based powder to achieve their whiter-than-white complexions, giving new meaning to the term "killer beauty." What is a master's degree, compared to this delicious information?

I do not subscribe to these magazines, partly because I entertain the idea that I can take them or leave them—like an alcoholic, I think, *I can quit whenever I want!*—and partly because it is so much more exciting, a real time-consuming *project,* to get dressed, go out, buy them, and bring them home. Like hunting—the satisfaction of slaying what I need to sustain me.

There are side effects, however. It's possible to gorge too thoroughly on beauty tips. This happens when I devour more than one magazine at once, or when I pour over every word of an extra-thick, phone-book-sized "Special Beauty Issue" packed with prettily packaged products. Midway through one of these tomes, I have a dull headache; next comes an uneasy, jumpy feeling. Still I plunge ahead, compelled to finish it. I admire the woman who can casually pick up a copy of *Glamour* on her lunch hour, flip through it while she eats, then tuck it back into her desk drawer until the next day. Folding pages, making lists, I become twitchy with need. I *must* have these products. Now. Yesterday. How soon can I get to the store, and is it worth risking a panic attack for the victory of walking out with a little bag full of promise in my hand? What a sucker I am, to believe that the thrill of a new lipstick will last more than five minutes, will last past the peeling off of the tamper-proof plastic, the swiveling up of the little phallic tube out of its case? Another plummy red, similar to the one I bought last week. No: Buying the product and having it do not even begin to equal wanting it. I wonder how much of the allure is not so much the product itself but the prettiness of the model's face, the warm accessibility of her smile, the immediacy of her gaze? I hear that it's all so carefully calculated. The beauty-company executives test-market these ads in states like Ohio and Kansas, in search of the gullible, unjaded Everywoman who apparently resides somewhere in the Midwest. A city girl would be far too sophisticated for this hokum. Right? They're savvy, these marketing execs, probably in Armani suits. They survey these unsophisticated women, asking whether (circle one) they find the model to be A) accessible, B) intimidating, or C) appealing. Does she look like your best friend, or the girl you hated in high school? How clever and manipulative those advertisers are! I am on to them. And yet, a part of me thinks, *I will look like her when I use this product. I will feel the joy/sexiness/ confidence I see in her air-brushed gaze.* It's fill-in-the-blank advertising, and I am a willing blank needing to be filled.

Back when I was in college, when I had places to be and things to do and people to see, the magazines were just a welcome distraction. A treat. They were not life and death. They were a Band-Aid for a bad day. Lately, though, they feel more like pressing a bit of gauze over a gushing wound.

I've become a tiny flame, straining toward the oxygen of any brief thrill. To *think* is to become confused, distraught, riddled with insecurity. To act, however impulsively, is to dash over the abyss of self-doubt with only a minimum of pain. Like those people who chant and psych themselves up before running across hot coals or over broken glass, I am sure that if I don't think about it, I won't feel a thing.

Acting impulsively, I've also discovered, is in itself a kind of thrill, however short-lived. Forever in search of distraction, I have begun to practice recklessness in every area of my life. In the past two months, alone in my bathroom, I have dyed my hair every color from white-blonde to almost black. Last week, I had it lopped off into a spiky pixie one afternoon when I happened to pass a Supercuts on Santa Monica Boulevard. The rush of acting recklessly is like lighting matches; each tiny thrill burns brightly for only a few seconds before flaring out, and I am always searing my fingers. Watching the long strands of my hair fall to the floor, a terror caught in my throat. Still, of course, I forced a smile for the hairdresser, feigning delight at "the new me." I paid my ten dollars and then, feeling trapped and panicky at the finality of my new do, I went immediately from the salon to a wig store on Hollywood Boulevard. When the transvestite behind the counter wasn't looking, I slipped a long, streaky-blonde wig into my bag.

Acting impulsively is like dominoes. Each action knocks me further away from myself, until I feel I have become another person. My desire for change and distraction is like an undertow, and I've quit swimming at last and allowed myself to drift, carried away to wherever it might take me. I used to be a sweet, kind, conservative, well-bred girl; now, with my short hair and careless attitude I feel tough, aloof, brittle: Pat Benatar screeching out *love is a battlefield*. Will this persona stick? I'm trying on and discarding images of myself in a desperate attempt to see what fits. Which of these different "me's" will make me feel like . . . like *me?* The night before the party, I did something completely unlike the old Hope: I drank a bottle of my roommate Karen's white wine, then passed out on the bathroom floor. I hadn't planned on doing it. I knew that she was saving the wine for an evening with her boyfriend. But it was starting to get dark, and I could feel the familiar heavy pull start inside me. Sadness and despair: These are the shades that forever haunt me; I elude them however I can. I saw the bottle there and, suddenly, drinking it seemed like something to do.

I've only been really drunk once, in college, and the experience was so ghastly I have never repeated it. I've always feared alcohol and drugs, terrified as I am of losing control. I always knew that I was the sort of person who would become not relaxed but paranoid when high. Drugs were plentiful at USC, but only once had I smoked pot on the roof of the Phi Gamma Delta house with my boyfriend Hart. It was not the pleasant, mellow feeling Hart had promised; rather, after a couple of hits, I became convinced that the stars were shooting out of the sky like white-hot bullets at me. Terrified, I held up my hands to shield myself and thought, *But these are not my hands! They are attached to my body, but they are not my hands!* I thought of my fear of losing control as a weakness, a flaw, unlike my mother's brave ability to be reckless. Like my father, I am something of a rigid Puritan at heart, another quality about myself I long to discard, another reason to hate myself.

As I drank Karen's wine, I smoked one Marlboro after another. Smoking was another new habit, one which I did not really enjoy but with which I persisted with a grim determination. My roommates and I were not supposed to smoke in the apartment, but I decided that if I was drunk, I could not be held accountable for a silly rule. The drunker I got, the more careless I became with where I put out my cigarettes, until finally I just tossed the smoking butts onto the floor by my bed where they dwindled and died, leaving small wormy black scars on the hardwood. I was listening to music, and my mind felt like it was a plume of smoke, freed from the confines of my body. I vaguely remember crawling into the bathroom to throw up, then passing out with my cheek pressed to the welcome cool of the floor tiles. In the morning I awoke to Karen standing over me, her good-girl Southern-belle manners overcome with disgust. *I'm so sorry,* I mumbled, struggling to my feet, the pain in my head exploding like Fourth of July fireworks. *This isn't the kind of thing I usually do, it won't happen again, blah-blah-blah.* I could feel how glib and insincere I sounded.

Lately I have become aware of a bubbling anger inside me which directs itself toward my roommates. I think about their busy, seemingly happy lives and am filled with not envy, exactly, but a sharp stab of rage. Why can't I have those things that they have, all those normal life things? Why is it so hard for me to imagine having what they seem so effortlessly to have: normal lives, trusted friends, the ability to make it through a day without needing at least one nap? Instead, I have nothing, I do nothing, I see practically no one, and I am exhausted to boot. So I even things out a little. During the day, when no one is home, I go into their rooms and look through their stuff. I try on clothes, borrow CDs, look for clues. What book, if any, is on the nightstand? Are there condoms in the drawer? What secret letters might be hidden beneath a stack of neatly folded sweaters? I don't find much, certainly nothing that is scandalous or revealing, just evidence of the everyday active lives of three young women. I feel like a spirit, an unsettled shade, haunting the halls and corners of the apartment. I try to be very careful to put everything back where I found it, so there won't be evidence of a visitation. I doubt the girls would buy my story of a supernatural prowler.

I feel like I am once again in my grandparents' deadly quiet house, free to explore while my grandmother took a nap and the maid smoked cigarettes in front of the television playing Spanish soap operas in her tiny room. No one cared what I looked at or where I went, so long as I was quiet. I always brought a few toys from home with me but I soon tired of them. Exploring felt so much more like freedom; the freedom to be invisible. The house had no evidence of children, and I always left it that way, nothing broken, nothing left behind. Does it really matter, then, if I eat the last can of my roommate's tuna, or drink a bottle of her wine? They don't seem to notice, or if they notice, they don't say anything. I do not feel important enough to be of consequence to myself, let alone anyone else. Half the time I don't even feel *real*. I feel like a mere shadow, something too insubstantial to have an effect.

Inevitably, there are days when I simply cannot manufacture anything to distract me. I have exhausted my options, or else I am simply too tired, too bored, too lethargic to try. These are the days when the little pebble of dissatisfaction rattling around inside me becomes a shard of glass. I am cut to the quick with sudden aching despair, caught breathless with anxiety. I will do anything, *anything* to escape that feeling, *anything* to fill the emptiness.

No one in my family ever said the word *depression*. You might be "a bit down," or "a little on the blue side." Depression was for losers, lunatics, and weaklings. To be depressed was to admit failure. It was worse than being poor. In spite of overwhelming evidence to the contrary, my mother never said she was depressed. "Sad" was altogether different. Sad was what you felt when the dress you wanted at Neiman's was sold out. Depression was what people living in trailer parks felt, people with missing teeth who drank malt liquor from paper bags. My mother hid her Glenfiddich in the hall closet behind the tennis balls. There was one evening in the Napa Valley when the three of us went to dinner and my mother cried through all four courses. Tears fell into her avocado soup, her mixed baby greens with goat cheese, splashed onto her steak and into her crème brûlée. Because she did not want to make a scene, my mother was careful to keep her face from contorting. Instead, a weak but steady stream of tears dribbled out of the corners of her eyes, which she dabbed delicately every time the waiter approached. My father kept asking, "What's wrong, Virginia? What's wrong?" and she kept saying, "I don't know." It was a strained and awkward dinner, to say the least. I tried to keep eating, the mashed potatoes like Elmer's glue in my mouth. Later, in the car, my mother's crying abruptly stopped and she fell asleep. Stretched out on the backseat, I watched the prickly pattern of stars in the black, black sky.

In college, there was a girl in my sorority house who was in the habit of vomiting into Styrofoam cups and leaving them in the laundry room. For a long time no one knew who it was that was doing this. Her identity remained an infuriating mystery. The condemning attitude of the other girls shocked me. Rather than be sympathetic, they ranted about the offensiveness of what she was doing, as if she were not in pain but simply inconsiderate. Their reaction, I see now, was this: We are *all* hurting, so who are *you* to show what we so carefully hide? This girl, in revealing her pain, was uncovering the secret anxieties of all the other girls. Every little cup full of stinky vomit reminded them of just how close to the abyss they themselves walked. I feel, now, as if I understand that girl, what she was saying: *See how much I hurt. Do not look away. You feel it, too.* It turned out to be a girl no one suspected, a sweet, pretty blonde with a good GPA. She wasn't one of the most beautiful girls, or one of the smartest, or one of the most remarkable in any way. She was wholesome, friendly, cute. An all-American girl.

See how much I hurt.

When I can't sleep anymore, when there aren't any new magazines to distract me, when I can't possibly find another excuse to visit Dr. S—'s office, these are the days when despair settles into my body like fever, making my bones ache. I hurt, I ache, I writhe under the surface where no one can see. It is a misconception, the idea that depression is all in the head. It is a physical pain. It settles in the joints, making me feel prematurely old, making movement difficult. The hollows of my hips throb. I lie on my bed and try not to hurt. Despair rises off my body in waves like heat off a pavement. I rush back and forth to the mirror, checking, always checking; for what? To make sure I'm still there? Innocently enough, I'll think, *What if I had bigger lips?* I'll think about this for a while, play with the idea. And then something shifts, sometimes gradually, sometimes abruptly, and what was once just a thought slips into obsession. *What if I had bigger lips and a smaller nose?* I would be stunning, that's what. Or at least *closer* to stunning (it's another lie I tell myself, that I could possibly—that I *will*—one day look in the mirror and find myself beautiful). It's a riddle, really, with a trick answer: What would it take for me to be satisfied with my appearance? Answer: Everything. Nothing. Nothing and everything. There is no answer to be found, at least not in the mirror. Because the riddle I am really trying to solve is: What will it take to make me happy?

Mirror, mirror, on the wall, I just need larger breasts, that's all! I never think about what else I might want to change about myself, after I've changed this thing. I think: *Just this one little improvement and—happiness!* Heart pounding, suddenly swollen full of this new, miraculous hope, once again I'm full. Yes! Bigger breasts! All those other nagging, painful thoughts are neatly and swiftly eclipsed. All I can think about is how much better I'll look and how much more confident I'll feel with this *thing*, this change I want to make.

Carried along on this rush of excitement, I can pretend the thought of the surgery itself does not scare me. Even though I am afraid of blood, of pain, of what the doctors coyly call "discomfort" the way newscasters call advertisements "these messages," I tell myself that the only pain I'll feel will be mild, finite, easily controlled with Vicodin.

Maybe, if I weren't really so vain and squeamish, my obsession would have taken a more predictable form. I would stick a finger down my throat or dig a razor blade into my arm. Or step on the scale fifty times a day, count every calorie. Wouldn't all of these achieve the same purpose? Yes, but then again, my fascination with plastic surgery feels so right. It is the perfect modern-day affliction for a poor little rich girl like myself. How appropriate, that a Hathaway should choose a route to self-annihilation that is elaborate, expensive, and essentially passive. I'm not brave enough to carve myself up in private; I've got to pay someone else to do it.

What if I had bigger breasts?

After the initial thought, as I said, obsession begins to take over. Something changes, and it's no longer that I just *want* to have this surgery, but that I *must* do it. I am *compelled* to go through with it. It becomes a personal mission, a test of my resolve. I *must* fix this flaw, or improve this feature, because once discovered, it will haunt and disturb me until I do. Sort of like those trick birthday candles: You think you've extinguished them with a big breath, but then they keep flaring up again. And here is the beauty, so to speak, of my little fixation: Caught up in the thought of a newer, better me, all my other worries are conveniently eclipsed. Because, after all, what are the prosaic concerns of daily life, compared to a risky, potentially life-threatening surgery?

CHAPTER 14

We meet at a small café near the beach in Venice.

Hank, I notice, wears a gold ring on the third finger of his left hand. It isn't a wedding band, but rather some sort of rodeo scene, a bulky depiction of bucking horse and rider. I wonder if he wears Stetson cologne.

He talks on and on about the movie he's filming with Dolph Lundgren, while I lick my upper lip, hoping the paint and spackle are still in place. The truth is, my upper lip has collapsed like a failed soufflé. The middle part is permanently full from the surgery, but without the Gore-Tex for balance, each side slumps somewhat unevenly. It's not noticeable unless you are really close to my face, and even then one might just think I was born this way, with a slightly odd-shaped upper lip. If I trace the outline with lip pencil and fill it in with gloss, it isn't noticeable at all. Besides which, Hank is too busy staring at my breasts to notice my mouth.

Starving, I order a hamburger, medium-rare, and a glass of red wine and then a hot fudge sundae. The emptiness I feel around Hank makes me want to fill myself up, makes me grateful for the surge of appetite. Hank drinks iced coffee after iced coffee. He cannot eat anything because of his movie, which requires that he look good in a Speedo. He must consume only diuretics, he says, to get rid of his water weight. Hank is the movie villain to Dolph's hero, and tomorrow they are shooting a scene in which the two of them compete in an Olympian-style swimming event. As he talks, Hank's rodeo ring catches the light. "What a *great* time the cast and crew are having on the set every day!" he raves. What a *terrific* bunch of people they all are! It wasn't work, it was all fun and games. Just for a lark, the makeup artist had shaved his pubic hair into a heart! They were having *so* much fun.

After dinner, Hank suggests a walk on the beach. It is well lit, near a strip of shops and restaurants, so I agree. Hank offers me one of his unfiltered cigarettes, so strong it makes my head spin. Perhaps he mistakes my dizziness for a swoon, because he leans in to kiss me hard, pulling us both down onto the sand and guiding my hand to his crotch, which is already hard. I pull away, reminding him that this is a public beach.

"Don't be shy, baby," he says. "Everyone fucks on this beach. Look, there's someone over there." He points to a dark, vaguely human shape lying on the sand a hundred or so yards away.

"I think that's a homeless person in a sleeping bag," I say.

But Hank doesn't hear me, or else he doesn't care. He is determined to carry on, with or without my participation, and starts to touch himself.

Realizing that he is more interested in jerking off than raping me, I relax a little on the sand, feigning admiration while he performs what my mother always referred to as "self-abuse." The moon on the waves is actually quite pretty.

"You've excited me now," he says, his voice trembly with lust and accusation. His penis, poking out of his shorts, calls to mind ridiculous romance-novel hyperbole like "rigid tool" and "his manliness." I am not turned on by the sight of it. Nothing about Hank even remotely arouses me. I don't even feel revulsion. I just don't feel. When I was in high school, I knew who I liked and who I didn't like. Nothing killed a budding feeling of attraction on my part faster that a boy leaning over me on the dance floor and saying, "Did you know that your grandfather delivered me?"

"Oh, baby," Hank says. "Look how big it is."

I feel like Anne Boleyn; my head seems severed from my body. Thoughts clink about like tin soldiers—*I should be offended; get the hell out of here; what an asshole Hank is*—but I cannot join a thought to the force of a feeling. I sit there, stiff and immobile as a ventriloquist's hollow wooden dummy.

Hank's hand makes a slapping sound on his flesh. "I've got to finish what you started," he mutters. He groans, trying to make me touch him, and when I resist he continues without me. I look around anxiously for passersby, but there are none, save for the immobile shape on the sand. Maybe it's not a person sleeping after all, I think. Maybe it's a dead body.

"You're so beautiful," Hank says afterward. "You're so hot."

I struggle to my feet, numbly feeling like I've endured something. One of my legs has fallen asleep. Hank puts his hand on the small of my back as we walk, and gradually the jab of pins and needles dwindles to normal feeling.

At my car he tucks me inside, patting the tinny roof. "You're wonderful," he says, and there is something about this empty praise that feels familiar.

In my rearview mirror I watch Hank walk across the parking lot and wait at the street corner for the light to change. As I drive he becomes first a shadow, then a dark speck, then part of the night.

The small, bleak feeling inside me, though, does not vanish so quickly.

CHAPTER 15

I stop by Dr. S—'s office near the end of the day, hoping that I will be there when he comes out after seeing his last patient. Chatting with the nurse and the receptionist, with whom I've become friendly, I feel homey and secure. They invite me into the office area to wait for "Bob," who is doing a post-op on a buttock lift. Alana, the receptionist, has, lately, even dropped her aloof attitude around me. Together, we are chatty girlfriends. I find myself becoming the girl I was in college: sunny, self-deprecating, utterly likeable. It's a relief to sink into this familiar performance. Is this how Meg Ryan feels, when she does a romantic comedy? *Ah yes, I've done this before. I could do this in my sleep.* I bask in this feeling of acceptance, even if we are less like a family than the members of a fan club.

"Did you see the lips he did on that Bridget girl?" Alana says. "Unbelievable, beautiful lips. Like Michele Pfieffer's."

"What did he use?" Suddenly, I am flushed with excitement.

"Liquid silicone."

An alarm pings in my head. "Liquid silicone? Isn't that banned by the FDA?"

"It's not *banned,* exactly," Alana scolds. "It's not *illegal* or anything. It just isn't *approved* specifically for that purpose. But that's just our stupid country. In Europe they use it *all* the time."

"But if silicone breast implants are dangerous, how can liquid silicone be safe?"

"The whole breast implant thing is just a lot of unhappy women making noise, hoping to get a court settlement." Alana sniffs disdainfully, as Rena, the nurse, nods solemnly. "Besides, when Dr. S— injects the liquid silicone, he does it in tiny micro-droplets, so each one stays exactly where it should and nothing migrates anywhere, which is what happened when doctors used to inject whole syringe-fulls into people's cheeks and stuff."

"It ended up at their chin or in a lump in their necks, and they had to cut the whole thing out," Rena says. "*Not* a pretty picture."

When Dr. S— comes out, it is as if all the lights have gone on in a dark room. I turn my face up at him like a flower to the sun, feeling vulnerable, exposed, exquisite. I think, *A single moment of being seen can make up for a lifetime of invisibility.* "If you could do anything to me, what would you do?" I ask him.

Dr. S— looks at me and shrugs. "Not much," he says.

I always come to Dr. S—'s office in my very best clothes, clothes designed to impress, outfits my mother bought me in anticipation of the fabulous job interviews she thought I'd go on.

Dr. S—, I'll admit, is an appreciative audience. Once, I came to his office in sleek houndstooth-print pants and a white knit top, an ensemble befitting a junior executive. I could tell by the way his eyes lit up when he saw me that he approved of the way I looked, but it wasn't until after our appointment that he commented on it.

"This is *exactly* the way I like a woman to dress," Dr. S— said, putting his arm around me as we came out of the exam room where he had just checked my lip. There was the usual small group of staff and patients gathered in the office, and they all looked up at us. "What do you think?" he asked everyone and no one in particular. "Don't we make a good couple?"

The faces nodded, and I thought I would swoon with pleasure. We were at the door now, and I was looking forward to going home and basking in the afterglow of his praise.

"Has anyone ever told you, Hope," he said, "that you look *just* like a young Julie Andrews?"

"No." I tried to sound flattered, but my mind reeled. Julie Andrews? Was that a compliment?

"You really do look like her. Especially your profile."

A drumbeat of despair had started in my stomach. Of all the women I would have liked to have been compared to, Julie Andrews, even a young Julie Andrews, was not one that came to mind. "Thanks," I said.

All the way home, in my car, I felt like crying. When I got to the apartment, Anita was in the kitchen.

I couldn't contain myself. "Do you think Julie Andrews was pretty? I mean, when she was young?"

"Julie Andrews? Sure. In *The Sound of Music*? She was adorable."

"But was she *pretty?*"

Anita looked at me strangely. "She was pretty, yeah. In a cute, innocent sort of way. Why do you ask?'

"No reason. Someone just told me I look like her, that's all." I fussed with the coffeepot.

Anita cocked her head to one side, studying me. "I wouldn't have thought that, but now that you point it out, you do look a little like her."

"A little or a lot?"

"Um, a little, I guess. From a certain angle."

And what angle was that? I wondered, afraid to ask.

"Was it a guy who told you this?" Anita asked. "An older guy?"

"Yeah. He's about forty-five."

"Then it probably was meant as a compliment. Julie Andrews in her day was kind of a hottie."

A hottie? Julie Andrews in a dirndl skirt, singing in the Alps. Was this really a good thing? Hadn't she played a former *nun?* Oh, shit: I was going to obsess over this all afternoon.

Anita, I could tell, was trying not to laugh. "I mean, he did say a *young* Julie Andrews, right? It's not like he said, 'You look like Julie Andrews in *Victor/Victoria.*'"

"True," I said miserably.

"It *is* a compliment," Anita called over her shoulder, heading down the hall toward her room.

Was it? Maybe, yes, but Julie Andrews wasn't exactly Brigitte Bardot. She wasn't even Linda Evans. She was, as far as I was concerned, fairly far down the list of knock-out gorgeous women. I wanted Dr. S— to see me as an irresistible sexpot, not a yodeling governess.

Worse, though, are the times when he turns the sunshine of his attention on another patient. The next time I am in the office, he shatters my precarious sense of well-being by admiring a dark-haired girl of about eighteen. She must be a new patient; I've never seen her there before, and I am in the office enough to recognize all of the regular clients. The two of them are coming out of an exam room as I am coming in from the waiting area.

"She looks *just* like a girl I dated in college," Dr. S— is saying. "She was the heir to a bubble gum fortune."

He puts his arm around the girl's slim shoulders and she blooms under his attention, leaning into him a little. Dr. S— shakes his head ruefully, thinking about what he missed out on. "Can you believe it?" he says. "A bubble gum fortune."

Watching them together, I feel flayed.

One afternoon, I allow Dr. S— to inject a syringe full of bovine collagen into my upper lip, to correct the "asymmetry" which previous procedures have produced. Beneath a quadrant of white lights, like a spaceship descending upon me, I close my eyes as he injects numbing lidocaine into both sides of my face, between the bridge of my nose and my cheekbone, where the central nerves of the face run. My eyes water, a tingle creeps up either side of my nose toward my eyes, but I do not go numb. Dr. S— massages the area to encourage the spread of the lidocaine; still, nothing. My lips retain full sensation. He administers a second and third injection; this time, tears run down my cheeks and soak into the collar of my shirt.

"Numb yet?" he asks.

I shake my head.

Dr. S— decides to "give it a few minutes," during which he leaves to see another patient. I keep tapping and pinching my lip, but there is not even the slightest lessening of sensation.

Dr. S— returns. He is puzzled. "I'll give you another injection," he says. "And if this doesn't work, you're a horse." This time, he jabs the needle into my flesh with unusual force. My entire nose goes numb, but the numbness does not spread downward to my lip.

Dr. S—, flummoxed, says he has never had this happen before.

"Is it possible," I ask, "that my cheek implants are blocking the nerve?"

"I didn't think of that," Dr. S— says. "Yes, that's possible. In fact, that must be it."

You didn't *think* of that? I want to scream. It's written right on my chart! He does not apologize for his oversight, or for making me endure six unnecessary shots. He refills the syringe with lidocaine, then bends over me once again. "This will be more painful," he says flatly, jabbing the area between my upper lip and my nose. "Don't move," he admonishes me, when my body jolts with pain like someone in the electric chair. "If you move, you'll risk hurting both of us."

Finally, after I am numb, he injects, little by little, a syringe full of collagen into my lip, stopping often to stand back and appraise his work. When we are done, he says approvingly, "That is some lip." He hands me a mirror and I look at my reflection. My face is distorted from the multiple injections of lidocaine, and my lifeless upper lip is stiff and immobile, like a trout's gaping mouth. He hands me a tissue so that I can wipe away the trails of mascara which my tears left on my cheeks. I lick the tissue and run it over my face, but there are a couple of dark smudges that will not budge, no matter how hard I rub at them. Dr. S—, noticing my efforts, says, "Oh, that's where I hit a blood vessel. You'll have a black eye."

Sure enough, by the time I leave his office the skin beneath my right eye is purplish and swollen. I don't have any concealer with me, so I put on sunglasses to hide my shiner.

By that evening, it looks as if I've been punched.

The black eye lasts for a week. It takes all my skill to disguise it with makeup; still, my beat-up face draws stares when I go out, the sort of glances in which people look, look again, then look quickly away.

I wonder, throughout the week, whether Dr. S— thinks of me with my black eye. I wonder if he gives even a moment's thought to the bruise I wear, or the effort it takes to conceal it.

Two weeks after the collagen injection, I see Dr. S— again. My black eye is gone, and my upper lip is, in fact, alluringly full and well-balanced to my lower one. As always, the anticipation of our meeting rings in my head as I wait for him in the exam room. Will he be in a rush today? How can I prolong our time together?

"Hope." The sight of Dr. S— in the doorway, smiling at me, makes me want to burst into tears the way people in airports do when they see their loved ones stepping off the plane. "My goodness, look at you," he says. "You're a vision."

I want to embrace him, but instead I murmur, demurely, "Thank you."

"So how do you like your result?"

I wonder if he means the result of the collagen injections, or "my result" in a more general sense, encompassing all the procedures he's performed on me. "My lip looks good," I say. "And I liked the lift, but . . . I think my eyes are starting to look the way they did before." In fact, they look exactly the way they did before. The slight exotic uptilt has gone away, and I am back to looking like the girl next door. Like Julie Andrews. More disturbingly, I have two hairless scars, about two inches long and a half-inch wide, on each side of my head. I can't wear a ponytail, or they will show. I will have to hide them for the rest of my life.

"Some loosening of the result is inevitable," Dr. S— says breezily. "Besides which, subtlety is the goal."

I almost laugh. *Subtlety?* I think. *In your office?* I cannot help but see the irony of this. "Yes," I say. "Of course. Subtlety."

"You know, Hope, there's something I tell all my patients." Dr. S— sits down on the little stool, and my heart lurches with longing at the prospect of a few more minutes together. "I like to say that the relationship between patient and surgeon is similar to the relationship between patient and therapist. You tell me where you want to get to, and it's my job to help you get there."

"That's kind of a tall order," I say, half joking.

"We can do anything you want. There are so many ways . . ."

My mind wanders while he talks. *Anything I want? I want to be happy, or at least free of constant aching despair. I want to not have crippling anxiety. I want to be able to look in the mirror and not see only what I think is wrong and unattractive. I want to be loved. Can you do all that, Doctor?*

His voice is lulling as he continues to ramble on, pontificating, using his hands to illustrate a point in the air. I hear words—"doctor-patient trust," "prevention not correction," "early thirties." I'm not really listening until, with a final flourish, Dr. S—stands, dives forward to deliver a quick dry kiss to my cheek, and declares, "So I guess that's it, then."

No! I think. *So soon!*

His hand is on the doorknob.

"Doctor!"

That word.

Dr. S— turns back to me and I say it again, softer: "Doctor."

His eyes on me are expectant, attentive, waiting. "Yes?"

Once I say what I am about to say, giving voice to what I have been thinking about these past weeks, there will be no turning back. The wheels will be set in motion, and a force stronger than myself will take over, the force of obsession. *I must have this surgery. I must I must I must.*

"Yes?" Dr. S—'s hand is still poised on the doorknob. He has other patients to see.

I think of his ad in the magazine, the blonde woman with the custardy breasts doing a back bend. I debate, but for only an instant.

"I was thinking about breast surgery." The words spill out of my mouth in a breathless rush, like a sob. "What do you think?"

Dr. S—'s hand slides off the doorknob. He crosses his arms over his chest, giving me his full attention. "Larger or smaller?" he asks.

His question startles me. Isn't it obvious? "Larger."

Dr. S—'s face lights up. Instantly he is back in the room, not just physically but emotionally. This is the moment I pray for. The door is closed, we are alone, there is no one else.

"Breasts are my specialty," he says. "Take off your shirt. Let's see what we have."

I shed my shirt and bra, utterly unself-conscious. His eyes on my naked skin raise goosebumps along my arms and stomach. I put my arms at my sides, my exposed breasts like offerings.

Dr. S— looks from my face to my breasts. A smile spreads slowly across his mouth. My nipples pucker, then stiffen under his gaze. Dr. S— nods his head, looking slowly from one breast to the other. He reaches out to cup each breast in his hand, as if weighing it in his palm. It is all I can do not to cry out.

"The right one is a little bigger than the left," he says. "But on the whole, you've got very nice breasts."

I feel deflated. How can he not feel the heat, the intimacy of this moment? How can he not take everything I have to give him?

"After the surgery, though, you'll have traffic-stopping breasts."

After the surgery? I think, startled. I haven't decided yet. I told him I was *thinking* about larger breasts. I didn't say I would do it.

"Your skin has wonderful elasticity." Dr. S—'s voice is husky, but for me, the moment is lost. "You're very lucky, Hope. With your young skin and your frame, you can carry off a very large implant."

"I don't know if I would want *very* large breasts." My heart beats so hard he must be able to see it through the pale sheath of my skin. I can't tell if I am enraged or insulted or simply stung by what feels like his rejection. "I haven't even given it that much th—"

"It's a *won*derful decision," he says. "You'll absolutely *love* your result, I promise. You won't have any regrets."

I recall, in college, a boyfriend who praised my breasts as perfect. I imagine myself running down La Cienega with my new, fake breasts in a tiny white bikini, like Pamela Anderson, cars crashing into lightposts.

"The thing is . . . I, uh . . . I really haven't given it enough thought. I have to think about it."

Disappointment—or is it some darker emotion?—clouds Dr. S—'s face. "Take your time," he says unconvincingly. He is once again poised at the door. He has other patients waiting to see him. Patients quicker to make a decision than me, more sure of what they want. I cannot take up any more of his time. "Let me know what you decide," he says, without feeling.

"It's just . . . I'm afraid that . . ."

"Yes?" Dr. S— is annoyed now.

"I just don't want to become some kind of plastic surgery junkie."

"*Please.*" Dr. S—'s staccato laugh echoes so shrilly in the little room, I can feel it in my teeth. "'Plastic surgery junkie'? Please. You have no idea."

"What do you mean?"

"What I mean is, talk to me when you're on your fourth nose

job. Or when I'm liposuctioning your thighs for the third time because you think I *missed a tiny bump.*"

His eyes are hard and bright. Something unfamiliar twists inside me, something I haven't felt before in his presence.

"Anyway, Hope, let me know what you decide about your breasts." Abruptly the angry tone is gone, and Dr. S— is once again the affable physician-magician, ready to make me into whoever I want to be. "Don't be a stranger," he says, winking. "I'm always here for you."

In the elevator I realize what it is I feel for Dr. S—: dislike, or its darker cousin, revulsion. It's what I feel sometimes during my encounters with Hank, when I feel at all. I am terrified of my own anger, which I sense is so strong that it must be muffled with confusion and static. Perhaps if I could face, even a little, my own deep agony, I might be able to stop this slow-motion train wreck that is my life. But like the ninety-pound bulimic sticking her finger down her throat as she sobs, or the alcoholic downing the drink he knows will make him black out, my sense of dread is not so great as my despair, a force that hurtles me toward oblivion, toward disaster.

CHAPTER 16

In the Food section of *Vogue* magazine, there is an article about cooking the perfect lobster. But I am not as interested in the virtues of boiling versus grilling as I am in a short description of the lobsters' mating habits, which seem to bear a similarity to those of myself and Hank:

In the summer, just before she molts, the female lobster enters the dominant male's shelter. They then engage in a boxing ritual which may last for several minutes, during which the female may become violent. Before molting, the female faces the male and rests her claws on his body. There is much touching of antennae. Then her carapace, her main body shell, splits free from her tail, and she pulls herself out. She is then completely vulnerable. She can hardly stand on her own legs. The male then stands over the female, holding himself up by his claws and tail, and turns her over gently with his ten legs. Mating lasts between eight seconds and a minute. He then stands guard over her for a week while eating her discarded shell. Afterward the female leaves, burying herself in the sand until her shell is again hard enough to offer protection.

Hank has an almost hypnotic effect on me. When he calls, wanting to talk dirty, I do not hang up on him. When he appears at my door, I let him in. When he wants to fuck me without a condom, I let him. I am playing with fire, and I know it, but I am, it seems, powerless to stop it. There is always that first moment when I think I will refuse, turn him away, hang up. When I think I will find my voice and deny him. But my resolve crumbles, a crumbling that becomes a landslide of complete acquiescence. Increasingly reckless, I make no distinction between little risks and huge ones. I give no more deliberation to having unprotected sex with Hank than I do to cutting my hair short. I used to think that there was something liberating in acting recklessly, the way my mother acted, but I see, now, that it is not about freedom but about enslavement. It is about helplessness. I saw a glamor in my mother's pain but there was, for her, nothing indulgent about it. What she was surrendering to was beyond her control. It was not a sumptuous giving over to but a mute giving in. I have felt the thrill of certain acts of recklessness—the times in Dr. S—'s office when I push the doubt out of my mind and agree to a procedure. There is a sort of thrill of defiance in that moment which I say to myself, *So what, who cares, I won't think about it. Screw common sense and reason, screw* you. But who am I screwing, really? My recklessness is more like carelessness. It is not thrilling. It is grim and angry and full of an unexpressed violence.

There is, from the start, so much mute rage in my encounters with Hank. I tell myself that what we are having is just a casual affair, but it is so much more than that. Psychologists say that we re-create, as adults, painful situations from our childhood in an unconscious effort to better resolve them. With Hank, I unknowingly re-create every situation in which I was unseen, unheard, defined by other people's ideas of me as a predatory, purely sexual being. I recreate the helpless rage of Hugh's advances, my silence in the face of my mother's accusations that I seduced my father. I subject myself to Hank's advances and feel the same sinking anger, the same flattening helplessness. It is a raping of all my faculties, the only defense against which is a forced numbness. The anger, though, is always there; it does not go away. I want to hurt someone, to damage them irreparably, and because the force of my anger terrifies me, I turn it upon myself.

After our first encounters, Hank isn't interested in normal, straightforward sex. He'd rather talk about it while jerking off. Sometimes, he doesn't even want to come, just wants to caress himself. He is fascinated by the sight of his own rising penis. He brings over pornographic films and we watch them together. I even make popcorn. How amazing, Hank says, how *cute,* really, that at twenty-three I have never seen a porno movie! I can see that Hank becomes interesting to himself in new ways when he is around me. He fancies himself the Professor to my Eliza Doolittle, ready to school me up in smut. I have always been a good student. My pornographic experience was characteristically rather effete: I had a copy of *Delta of Venus,* which I'd read in college, feeling very sophisticated and Left Bank. After the films, which we watch, strangely enough, fully clothed, eating popcorn, he quizzes me as to what I thought of them.

I think about this with an intellectual detachment. "I didn't know there'd be so many close-ups," I say.

"What did you think of the red-haired woman?" Hank asks. "Wasn't she incredible?"

I reflect on this like I'm back in English class, being asked about the motivations of Madame Bovary. "It was something," I say, "the way she could suck her own tit."

"Didn't she have a nice pussy?"

Gee, I hadn't really thought about it. But now that he asks, "Yes. It *was* kind of nice, neat and compact. Her clitoris looked sort of like a stunted and frostbitten bud. Very Georgia O'Keeffe."

Hank isn't interested in my stunning metaphors. On another day, he says, "I have plans for you." His plan is that he wants me to dominate him. He's been hinting at it for weeks, and I've deliberately ignored him. I fear I am not assertive enough to give commands. Then, one day, perhaps no longer able to contain himself, he throws himself on my bedroom floor, naked and cowering, and cries, "Mistress! Don't hurt me!"

This is something I've only read about. Dungeons, leather, whips, and chains. Still, I am sure I can get the hang of it. It is something to do, at least, isn't it, a tiny hurdle to overcome? If all the surgeries have not changed me into someone else, perhaps being with Hank will. I tell myself that I am being daring and adventurous, exploring a world which my sheltered upbringing never hinted at. I am becoming blasé and cosmopolitan. I tell myself that the affair with Hank, what I call my "aloof" response to him, is a kind of progress. By holding something back, I am in control, as safely unfeeling as a robot. I am narrating my own gritty documentary, about the kind of affair a single girl has in Los Angeles, with an actor who will never be a movie star. With Hank I almost fool myself into believing that I am someone entirely different than the girl I used to be.

I stand over him in my bra and panties and my black leather boots. "Get down, scum!" I snarl.

Instead of cracking up with laughter, as I half expect him to, Hank hurls himself on the floor, cowering at my feet.

I feel a rush of power. "Lick my boots!" I command.

Hank whimpers with delight, running his tongue over my boots. "Stupid pig!" I say. "Bad, bad boy!" I suppose I ought to come up with something dirtier, or more imaginative, but I can't seem to shake my hopeless sense of decorum. I realize, as I stand still for Hank to grovel at my feet, that I have unconsciously affected a debutante pose, hips squared, upper body turned slightly sideways, one knee bent slightly.

I brace the heel of my boot against Hank's shoulder. "Didn't you hear me?" I yell at him. "I said to *lick my boot!*"

Hank obliges, slurping at my sole like an eager puppy. I think about where I walked earlier that day, wearing the same boots: down Larchmont Boulevard, a street frequented by people with dogs. Sanitation overrules erotica. Even Hank doesn't deserve a mouthful of dog shit, though he might even like it.

"Get up slave," I say. "On your knees."

"Mistress!" he cries.

I dig my heel into his shoulder, but something stops me from going further, from drawing blood. If our relationship spills over into actual violence, how many more areas of my life will topple like dominoes, revealing their unacknowledged brutality?

Hank sometimes comes to me smelling of patchouli or lavender, and I imagine him in the arms of some fragrant hippie girl. I suspect that my apartment is just one of several places where he stops for sex during the course of a day. I tell myself that I get a kind of perverse pleasure out of our encounters. A pleasure that is purely cerebral, safe and sound in my head. The fact that I can treat Hank as cavalierly as he treats me is comforting. It feels like evening a score. When I run my hands over his perfectly sculpted body and feel nothing more than if I caressed cold marble, it's as if I've gained back a measure of what I've lost.

Though I tell myself that I am pretending to be someone else when I am with Hank, I sometimes think that I am not pretending at all. Perhaps this *slut,* this *whore* is the real me. I am not so much becoming as succumbing. I've always *felt* wrong, bad, unworthy. That girl in the white gown, waltzing blithely around a ballroom; who was she? She was a fabrication. She was Cinderella with her head up her ass. What a relief it is to toss her away at last like a tired old Halloween costume. The fact that Hank treats me like someone worthless and disposable feels *right.* I'm accepting a punishment I've had coming all my life, the fulfillment of my aunt Helen's long-ago words in the kitchen: You'll get just what you deserve. I've adopted a stray cat, a large orange tom I call Henry Miller. When Hank and I are on the bed together, Henry watches us warily from a corner of the room, his large yellow eyes full of, I think, contempt.

To Anita, my roommate, I am able to adopt a startling flippancy when describing my relationship with Hank. *I'm glad to have someone, like, who makes all the effort*, I say, *even if the effort consists mainly of taking off his pants.* She wonders why I don't mind how one-sided our relationship is: I don't care to know his address; it doesn't upset me when he mutters something vague about how we can't go to his place because of some "construction" his landlord is doing. I tell Anita that I turn off my mind along with my body during my encounters with Hank, and so experience a kind of escape. It occurs to me that what I'm describing is, perhaps, what I've been searching for all my life: a not-caring. With my mother, my father, with boyfriends, with Dr. S——, I always felt like the weaker one, the one who wanted, the one who pined for *more*. I tell Anita that Hank is no more than a sexual object to me, when the truth is I am the one who is objectified, unseen, unheard, dismissed as purely sexual. It is not victory I've achieved but a familiar defeat.

CHAPTER 17

I read this about suicidal people: Sometimes, they decide to finally go through with it simply because they can't stand that little voice in their head anymore telling them to *do it, do it*. They just want to stop the noise. The same is true for other compulsives. Self-mutilators, hair pullers: Sooner or later, they give in to that little nagging voice.

Do it, do it, do it. This is the chant I hear in my head, but it's not telling me to kill myself or to cut myself or to pull out my hair strand by strand. It's telling me that this thing about my appearance, this one thing I've focused on and can't stop thinking about, *I must change this thing.* I can't tell anymore if I actually *want* bigger breasts, or if I simply want to stop obsessing about them. I can't think about anything else.

I stop by Dr. S—'s office and ask Alana to schedule the surgery for four weeks from now. I tell myself that this will leave me plenty of time to back out.

Dr. S— stops by Alana's desk while I am making my appointment. He is thrilled, of course, with my decision. "You absolutely will not regret this," he says. "But then, I'm a breast man." He tells me he just did the breasts of an exotic dancer, and she has since tripled her income.

"That's great," I say, even though this is not a category into which I wish to be placed. It is not snobbism that makes me shudder at the thought of slinking around a pole, wearing only a G-string, my newly inflated, traffic-stopping breasts holding the glassy stares of a hundred anonymous men. There is, to me, something threatening about being the object of such frank sexual desire. Having been accused myself of being a seductress, I shiver at the thought of that empty attention. I do not want to dangle myself tantalizingly over the hungry mouths of men. What I crave is something more immediate, more intimate, more like love.

What I haven't considered is the fact that Dr. S— requires a deposit of one half the total cost of the operation, which is six thousand dollars. He says that this is standard procedure, that he always requires a deposit for major surgeries like this, which he calls "a breast job."

"Partial payment is required *up front,* heh heh," he says. "So to speak!"

He has to order the implants from Dow Corning, a company which I know manufactures all kinds of plastic parts. It makes me think of putting together a toy: *Look for Dr. S—'s creations in the Large Dolls aisle!*

I do not have room left on any of my Visa cards for a three-thousand-dollar charge. I've been taking cash advances to pay my rent and buy groceries. I open my wallet and stare into it, at the various collection of receipts and miscellaneous bits of paper upon which I've scribbled things that seemed important enough to write down. I stare at this flotsam and jetsam as if it will yield up an answer as to how I am going to pay for this surgery.

And then, miraculously, it does.

Poking up from a forgotten pocket is the mint-green edge of an American Express card my father gave me when I went off to Berkeley. It was, he said, to be used only for emergencies. I had charged school books on it, some clothes. I had forgotten I even had it.

I pull out the card with a flourish, like a magician pulling a rabbit from a hat. I hand the card to Alana, feeling a rush of victory. But wait: Doesn't American Express need to be paid each month? In full, up front, as Dr. S— would say? Will the bill still go to my father? And if it does, will he pay it?

As Alana's manicured hand closes over the thin rectangle of plastic, the worry pounds in my head. Will the bill come in after I've had the surgery, or before? What if the American Express people call my father?

Dr. S— goes off to see a patient, and Alana slides the card through the machine. She waits, then punches numbers into the machine, knitting her brow.

"It's telling me I need to call the eight-hundred number," she says.

Oh no, I think. *This is it. I've been caught. It's all over.* My heart sinks, my stomach plunges with disappointment.

"Hope? The credit card company wants to speak to you in person." Alana holds out the phone to me.

"Hello?" My hand trembles as I hold the phone to my ear. I listen as the clipped and efficient male voice at the other end asks if this is, indeed, Miss Hope Hathaway. I say that it is. Can I tell him my social security number, my mother's maiden name? I do, wondering if this is how they stall a criminal on the phone while the police are called. He then apologizes for the "inconvenience" of having to call me, but it's just that my card has been inactive for so long, and now this major charge comes along. They just need to make sure it's not fraud, that's all. Could I confirm for them that I, Hope Hathaway, authorize them to pay Doctor Bob S—, A Medical Corporation, the amount of six thousand dollars?

I realize, then, that Alana has charged the full amount of the surgery on the card. I am both shocked and relieved at this, and hesitate only a moment before taking my solemn vow.

"I do," I say.

On the way back to my apartment, stuck in traffic, random thoughts swirl around in my head. I think about how I have always hated roller coasters. Just seeing one on television makes my palms sweat with dread. And yet, as a child, I always forced myself to go on them. What I wanted was the particular thrill I felt when I stepped *off* the ride, a combination of relief and joy and the adrenaline rush of fear.

There was one roller coaster that particularly terrified me, the Space Mountain ride at Disneyland. I remember going on it with my father when I was about eleven or so. My mother hated roller coasters, so this was an opportunity for the two of us to do something together. I liked this part of roller coasters, too, the fact that I got to be alone with my father, something my mother so rarely allowed. In the Space Mountain line, I remember thinking, *This is one thing that she is afraid of doing, and I am going to do it. I am braver than her, bolder, more daring.* I remember holding my father's hand as we wound around in the line, waiting our turn. The line was long; it was a summer weekend. After inching along for about half an hour, there was a sign that read, in large ominous black letters, IF YOU DO NOT WISH TO GO ON THIS RIDE, YOU SHOULD LEAVE NOW. My father looked down at me and I squeezed his hand, walking forward, feeling brave. At a certain point the line entered a darkish, space-themed building where the actual roller coaster was. There was a futuristic soundtrack of whooshing comet sounds and other mysterious, terrifying, high-speed space noises. A little further on, there was another sign. This one was on a door. It said: THIS IS YOUR LAST CHANCE NOT TO GO ON THIS RIDE. LEAVE NOW. It felt like a dare. I thought, *Like hell I'm going to leave now.*

It was deliberately dark, to approximate being in deepest space. We were close enough to hear the screams of the people on the ride, even though we couldn't see them. I'd dropped my father's hand, embarrassed by how sweaty mine was, and shuffled along, stiff with fear. *Ice cream with caramel sauce,* I thought. *Cotton candy, cracker jacks, corn dogs. A Mickey Mouse cap with my name stitched on it in big scrolling letters.* If I could get through this ride, I could have these.

Then, suddenly, we were at the front of the line, an impatient crush of people behind us. An attendant was gesturing me into the roller coaster car. My father was already strapped in, waiting for me.

When the ride was over, I was shaking so hard my father had to lift me out. My head held a tremor that would not go away. I walked mechanically down the ramp and out into the sunlight, my father's big hand cupping my shoulder. I felt like I might throw up. And yet, I felt . . . *alive.* That feeling, of every cell in my body vibrating with life, was worth all the anguish. The world was in Technicolor again. The bright sun, the musical splashing of a fountain, the taste of vanilla ice cream were all so much more intense, so profound. Joy felt purer. I felt grateful and elated and alive. I remember thinking that if I could live in that intensity all the time, I would be happy.

Now, in my car, I see the similarity between the little girl I was and the woman I am now. We each seek the same thing: excitement, connection, an escape from the mundane. The stakes are higher now; it is an operating table instead of a roller coaster car that I am climbing onto. But I am still the same. I am the same girl who inched along in the theme park line, breathless with fear, my eye fixed on the signs that offered me an exit, knowing that I would not heed them.

CHAPTER 18

Hank has a part in a play, at a tiny theater off of Highland. It is a weird, abstract play in which everything is symbolic and nothing makes sense. His character is called The Strong Man, and he has to wear tights and a weight-lifter's suit and carry a Styrofoam barbell. The symbolism, I suppose, is that he is carrying the weight of the world. It is a terrible, silly play, and I feel a little embarrassed for Hank for being in it. Still, I sit through it twice, once by myself and the second time with my roommate Anita.

After the play, Anita and I wait outside the theater for Hank to come out. There is so much trash on the street here. Doesn't Hollywood ever clean its streets? Looking down, I spot a crumpled condom, cigarette butts, bits of clothing, papers, mysterious puddles. All this filth makes me want to stand on my tiptoes.

Seeing Anita, Hank instantly becomes his most magnetic, attentive self. For her part, Anita becomes coy and flirty, every bit the blushing Dairy Princess.

We talk for a few minutes about this and that, the Dolph Lundgren movie, which may not get a theatrical release, though Hank is
still optimistic. "Even if it goes straight to video," he says, "the
numbers in the overseas market will be enormous. Dolph is huge in
Japan."

"I'll bet," I say. "Especially considering most Japanese people are
about five-foot-five. Will they dub your voice?"

"Sure, I guess," he says. "Or maybe subtitles. Who knows?" He
makes it sound like the possibilities are endless.

We grab some coffee, then head back to the apartment. Anita
bids us good-night and goes to her room. Alone in my room with
Hank, I am surprised that he doesn't want to fool around. He says
he is having an allergic reaction to the rubber handle of the fake
barbell he has to carry in the play. Sure enough, his palms are a
livid red and peeling. "Every night I smear them with cortisone and
put gloves on," he says. "It's a fuckin' pain."

I yawn, hoping he'll take the hint. It's after midnight.

"So your roommate Anita," he says. "She's pretty hot."

"Uh-huh."

"I'd love to do a threesome with her."

"Sure," I say. "Dream on."

"I'm serious. Have you ever done a threesome?"

"No. And, to be honest, I really don't want to."

"It would be *so* hot. Think about it." Hank's hand automatically
reaches for his crotch. Oh shit, I think. I was hoping we were going
to call it a night.

"No, Hank."

"Of course, *you've* got the better body." He strokes my leg, perhaps thinking I'm jealous, or that he can persuade me with flattery.
"I've always fantasized about doing it with a fat girl."

"No, Hank. Forget it. You can fantasize all you want, but I'm
not doing a threesome. And as for Anita, she's my friend, okay?
Leave her alone. And stop referring to her as 'a fat girl.' "

He looks at me and there is a strange hardness in his eyes.
Something flashes there: shock, rage; I have done the unthinkable.

I have denied him. Almost instantly the look is gone, and he is playful again, tweaking my nipple through my shirt, tugging at my hair, hopping up and down to wake himself up for the drive home. When he leaves, he says, "Bye, Gorgeous."

But that look he gave me lingers in my mind. It is a look I've seen once before, weeks earlier, on one of the few occasions when we met in public, at a café. It had been at my insistence that we meet there. Hank never suggested we meet in public. I suspect that he has a wife or girlfriend tucked away somewhere and is concerned someone might see us. This thought didn't affect me either way. Still, I felt like asserting some authority over him, so I told him that if he wanted to see me, we had to meet where I said.

Hank had arrived somewhat late, and out of breath. Maybe he was nervous. He wore the same clothes he always wore, a black T-shirt and a charcoal blazer and dark trousers and big black shoes. Gangster clothes. I wondered if this was a look his agent encouraged.

"You look incredible," he said. This was promising; usually Hank only doled out compliments when he had his penis in his hand. Perhaps meeting him outside of my bedroom had been a good idea.

"Thanks," I said. He had a large, angry pimple on his cheek, badly disguised with a bit of makeup. Makeup! This made me feel like laughing, this little bit of obvious vanity. I, too, had a pimple on my forehead I'd taken pains to cover up. I liked how I felt: more powerful, in control of things. Things felt more *even*. The opposite of how it was when we were in my apartment.

Hank wanted to go right to my place, claiming he had an audition later that afternoon. But I felt a spiteful glee, determined to be the one in charge of things for a change. I decided to string him along.

"Let me drink my coffee first," I said. I noticed his T-shirt was on backward; the tag was in the front. It seemed like the kind of thing he might have taken the time to notice, before going to an audition. What did he do, dress in the car?

When I'd finished the coffee, I said, "I just have to pick up something at the pet store." Hank came with me as I took my time picking out a new litter box for Henry Miller, the biggest one they had, with a huge plastic cover and a filtered ventilation system.

"Would you carry it for me?" I asked him sweetly. He had to say yes, of course. My car was several blocks away, and he lugged the big contraption, sweating, tripping once over a curb. At the car, I thwarted him again.

"I'm not feeling well," I said. "Let's call it a day."

Hank seemed to make a great effort at controlling his frustration. He loomed over me, his elbow resting on the roof of the car so that my head fit in the crook of his arm, almost a wrestling hold. There was a perceptible tightening in the muscles around his eyes and jaw. Mixed with the exhaust of passing cars, his cologne smelled vaguely like Lysol. As he leaned over me, I realized how much bigger and stronger he was; if he wanted, he could easily force me into the car. Something in his look told me that this was exactly what he wanted me to consider.

It occurred to me that maybe this was what I wanted from Hank: a reaction. Any reaction. Something that would at least tell me I was on the radar. Even if it was a slap, it would be something.

Then, abruptly, he stepped back, giving me his familiar crooked smile. It was the smile of a movie villain—knowing, dastardly. It occurred to me that maybe I was unconsciously trying to raise the stakes of our relationship, to increase the danger and thus the thrill. What would happen if I pushed Hank too far? Would he hurt me?

Kissing the good side of his face, I drove away. Hank stood there on the curb waving as I drove off down the block, like a forlorn child who's been dropped off by his mother on the first day of school. I felt badly, not for the way I'd treated Hank, because he hardly deserved to be treated well, but because I had invested time and energy in a pointless attempt to exert my superiority over someone whom I did not even care about.

At moments like this, my life, the whole sweeping scope of it, seemed so empty and hollow that I wanted to weep.

CHAPTER 19

I'm stirring a pot of Kraft macaroni and cheese on the stove when the doorbell rings.

I glance out the living room window; when I don't see Hank's car, I run down the stairs and open the front door.

"Hi, Hopie," my mother says. She is standing on my doorstep in a white linen pantsuit, holding a bouquet of assorted sweet-smelling flowers. "These are for you," she says, handing them to me.

"Thanks." I put my face into the cool blooms and am almost overcome by their heady scent. I am overcome, too, at the sight of my mother; or, I should say, at my reaction to seeing her. I had not thought that I missed her, but seeing her now makes me want to throw my arms around her neck and hug her. We are both tentative, though, standing a few feet apart, smiling wide, uncertain smiles at each other.

"So, this is your apartment," she says.

"Yes." Suddenly, I do not want her to come inside. I'm

ashamed of my messy room, my permanently unmade bed, the
stack of beauty magazines beside it as tall as the top of the mat-
tress. I don't want her to know I spend my days here, holed up in
humid self-examination.

"I came to take you out to lunch," my mother says. "That is, if
you're free. Can you go? I thought we'd go to The Petit Greek."

Can my mother possibly think that I would not want to go out
to lunch with her? Does she think I'm holding a grudge for the way
she left me after my surgery? I'm not, or if I was, it vanishes as I
look at her. Has *she* forgiven *me,* for what I did to myself?

"Sure," I say. "I'd love to. Can you give me a few minutes? I
have to turn off the stove. If you want to, you can—"

"I'll wait in the car, thanks. I have to make a call anyway."

In the kitchen, I fill a vase with water and put the flowers in. I
look into the pan at the eerily yellow cheese congealing around the
macaroni, then turn it over the trash. I put the pot in the sink and
fill it with hot soapy water to soak. I take a quick look in the mirror, feel the usual slash of disappointment, grab my purse, slip on
sandals, and sprint out the door.

Sliding into my mother's car, into the smell of leather, makes
me think of those long-ago afternoons when my grandmother
picked me up at school. My mother looks at me. "You look good,"
she says, and I know she is trying very hard not to scrutinize my
face. "I like your haircut. Very summery. The color, though, is a little bit . . . what do they call it? 'Goth'?"

"Yeah. I know." I touch at the short spikes. It's funny this focusing on my hair. The last time she saw me, my pummeled, post-op
face was almost unrecognizable. Both of us, I sense, want to avoid
that subject.

The Petit Greek is on busy Larchmont Boulevard, in the center
of Hancock Park. Locals call the block-long stretch of shops,
restaurants, and coffee houses "the Village." When I was growing
up, Larchmont Boulevard was a sleepy street frequented mostly by
the area residents. There was a general store with a tiny post office

at the back. There was one bank and a health food store called Quinn's. There was a pet store owned by two old women who were—shockingly!—lesbians. One of the women was known to be cranky, so that you quaked with fear when buying your goldfish. There was a single beauty shop, where the blue-haired, blue-blooded ladies tottered in weekly for a shampoo and set. There was a Baskin-Robbins, a dry cleaner, and a shop owned by an eccentric old woman who sold dolls and miniatures. Her name was Jean, and her store was called Jean's Accents. No one knew how she stayed in business. Her store window, with its tiny perfectly arranged scenes straight from the Victorian age, was always dusty. I once badgered my mother into buying me a doll for my dollhouse which I had admired in the window. My mother fussed over the price: fifty dollars. It was more than we could afford at the time. The doll, a miniature little girl, was dressed in lace with a matted mop of real hair on her head. Her arms, legs, and face were porcelain. I could fold her into the palm of my hand.

Today, Hancock Park has become trendy. People from Paramount Pictures Studio, which is a few blocks away on Melrose Avenue, frequent Larchmont Boulevard. Cafés spill their tables onto the sidewalk. The coffeehouse is overflowing with out-of-work-actor-types, lounging around in wicker chairs, smoking cigarettes, their dogs snoozing beside them. The general store is gone. There is a designer lingerie shop, a Kinko's, a Rite Aid, a yoga studio, and numerous hair salons. Going there, you are bound to see at least one celebrity, or at least a lot of people who look like celebrities. Parking has become atrocious. The pet store, the health food store: gone. All that remains of the "old" Larchmont is the Baskin-Robbins and, ironically, Jean's Accents.

After circling the block four times, we find a spot in front of Haas Hair Design. My mother looks at me, then gestures toward the hair salon. "Remember the ad?" she says.

"Yeah." Back in high school, I was the model for an ad that Haas ran in the *Larchmont Chronicle*. My mother kept a copy of that picture. I wonder now, with a twinge, whether I would feel something like regret, looking at it now.

It is, I will later learn, a hallmark of depression to see oneself as unattractive. Depression screenings, in fact, regularly include questions as to how the person taking the test feels about his or her own appearance. Depressed people judge their own looks much more harshly than do others. Though not aware of this psychological fact at the time, I am aware that, in spite of all the surgeries, I do not find myself at all attractive. In fact, I find myself much *less* attractive than before. It's a nasty cycle I'm stuck in: The more depressed I become, the more I dislike my looks; the more I dislike my looks, the more convinced I am that I must have more surgery; the more surgery I have, the more depressed I become . . . and on and on.

"Virginia!"

We are at the restaurant now. The owner, Dmitri, descends on my mother with kisses and murmurs of how wonderful she looks. We are seated immediately, at a large table, even though there is a line of people waiting.

After ordering iced teas, my mother reaches into her purse and pulls out an envelope. "This came for you," she says.

I take the envelope and my heart sinks. It is the bill from American Express.

"I opened it, actually," my mother says, looking at her hands, which are smoothing the tablecloth. "I shouldn't have, I'm sorry."

I nod, swallowing hard.

My mother takes a breath. "I don't know who this Bob S—, A Medical Corporation, is, or why you're paying him six thousand dollars. And, to be honest, I don't want to know."

Finally, she looks up at me.

"Your father and I have never taught you to be responsible with money, and I'm sorry about that. It was a mistake on our part. We wanted you to have everything, but apparently, everything is not enough." She gives a little nervous chuckle. "You know what I think about this surgery business. I can barely even say the word, it

hurts me so much to think about it. But you're an adult now, and
you can make your own decisions. However, your father and I are
not going to pay for them."

I nod again, my mouth dry.

"Having said that, we didn't think it was fair to just cut you off
at the bootstraps, you know? So here," she reaches into her purse
again, withdrawing another envelope, "this is to help you get on
your feet, but that's it. That's all we're going to give you."

I take the envelope, such a pure, unblemished white, and slide
my finger under the sealed flap. Inside is a check for a thousand
dollars.

"Thank you." I tuck it back in the envelope, then fold it into my
purse. I feel as if I might cry. She is right, I think: I'm responsible
for my own choices, even if they don't exactly feel like choices. My
parents shouldn't have to pay for them. But how the hell am I going to?

"So, now that that's over," my mother laughs, making a stab at
levity, "I have some big news to tell you."

"What?"

"Your father and I are moving out of Hancock Park."

"You are? Why? Where are you going?"

"Pasadena, probably. We've been looking. Our house is for
sale."

I'm speechless. The Hathaways have lived in Hancock Park forever. They are the very definition of "old guard." To be a Hathaway in Hancock Park is to be like royalty. Why would my mother
give that up?

"Something happened," she says. "Your father and I were held
up at gunpoint."

"Oh, my God. When? Are you all right? When did this happen?"

"A few weeks ago. It was on Sixth Street." My mother fiddles
with the napkin in her lap. "We were walking Princess."

"Oh. God." Princess is my parents' black Labrador retriever.

I wait for my mother to elaborate. When she doesn't I say, "Tell me how it happened, Mom. Exactly what happened."

"We were walking along," she says. "It was dark. Your father was a little ways behind me, waiting for Princess to do her business. I was speed-walking. This car pulled up alongside me. The door opened and a man jumped out. He pointed a gun at me."

"Jesus! What did you do?"

"I, well, I screamed, I think. Maybe the man asked for money or a wallet or something, I don't know. Your father came running. My legs collapsed and I fell down on the sidewalk."

"And then what? What did Dad do?"

My mother has twisted the napkin into a stiff little pyramid. "He turned around and started running in the other direction, to distract the guy."

"Wait a minute. Dad turned around and ran away? He didn't stay with you?"

My mother gives a little laugh, as if to say, *How can you be so silly?* But there is pain in her face. "I know, I know. I didn't get it at the time, either. It all happened so fast. But your father did it to distract the guy's attention from me."

"By *running away?*"

"Yes. Exactly."

I stir my iced tea, watch the little lemon seeds swirl and settle at the bottom of the glass. I can picture the scene: My mother screaming, my father running up to see what was wrong. Seeing the man with the gun. Seeing my mother fall to the ground. Then . . . running away?

"He didn't . . . the man didn't ask for Dad's wallet or anything?"

"Maybe. I don't know! It all happened so fast. Your father dropped the leash, that's all I remember. Then next thing I know, Princess is sniffing around my ankles, and the man with the gun gets back in the car and they drive off."

"Just like that?"

"Just like that. I think maybe they got confused, you know, this woman on the ground screaming, and the man—your father—running off down the street."

"Yeah, they probably didn't expect *that*. Holy shit, Mom."

"Yeah."

I don't know what to say, so I say: "You were lucky." All I can think of is my big, lanky, six-foot-six father, running away for dear life. Does my mother really believe his story about "distracting" the guy? Can she possibly believe this?

"Did you know," she says, "that criminals call Hancock Park 'the candy store'? That's what the police said. They said it's just getting worse and worse. Oh! Dmitri. That looks fan*tastic*." Dmitri puts the plate with my mother's salad on it in front of her, turning it just so, removing his hand with a flourish. The strips of chicken are laid out in a tic-tac-toe pattern.

The subject of the holdup is dropped.

The rest of the lunch passes quickly. My mother and I forfeit Dmitri's offer of espresso and baklava. Walking back to the car, we pass Jean's Accents. I say, "Can you believe she's still here?"

"I know," my mother says. "Unbelievable, isn't it? I don't know how she hangs on year after year."

When my mother's car slides up to the curb in front of my apartment, I do not want to get out. We embrace, at last, a quick, awkward hug managed over the gearshift but one that is long enough for me to sink my face into her neck and inhale the sweet, slightly yeasty scent of her skin, like good bread. Suddenly, I long to tell her everything: How very miserable I am. How, in six days, I will be lying on Dr. S—'s operating table, having my breasts enlarged. I want to cry to her, *Help me! Help me not to go through with this! Help me to not want to change anything else about myself!* But I know that her words, however reassuring, cannot take away the longing inside me, the pain that does not go away. There is only so long I can cry on her shoulder before I have to go back upstairs to my room and face my loneliness and my fear and my despair, my self.

That afternoon, I think about my parents' decision to move out of Hancock Park. How much easier it must be, to focus on moving, on the high crime rate of the area, than on the fact that my father ran away. Statistics are always safer than emotion.

It does not amaze me, the fact that my mother believes, or at least pretends to believe, my father's explanation of his cowardice. It is, I think, no different than my believing, despite evidence to the contrary, that if I fix the outside of myself, I will automatically fix the inside. We are each living with our private self-deceptions. The ability to believe them is encoded in our DNA like blonde hair and long, thin bones. But simply blaming my inheritance, my mother or my father or anyone else, is like believing that someone else will pay the American Express bill: a deception I can no longer indulge in.

CHAPTER 20

The countdown has begun: four days until surgery. I cannot take aspirin, drink alcohol, or smoke cigarettes. I have not told a single person about the surgery, not Hank, not my roommates, not my mother. If I die on Dr. S—'s operating table, he will not know who to call. There is so much guilt and shame and ambivalence in my decision; if I talk about the surgery, I'll have to acknowledge my feelings about it, and I cannot, will not, do that.

Time with Hank, though no more pleasurable than usual, at least helps keep my mind off my surgery. The encompassing numbness I feel in his presence leaks over to lessen the terror I feel.

He stops by after midnight, still made-up from the play, thick tan pancake smeared across his cheeks like war paint. We go to my room. All the roommates are asleep.

We don't fool around much anymore, Hank and I, and tonight is no exception. He talks dirty, I listen. His monologues, despite their pornographic content, have a lulling effect on me. When he's done talking, he jerks off.

Now he stands up, stretches, hoists his jeans up. With an exaggerated Schwartzenegger drawl, he says, "I'll be back."

I pick at my nails. I figure he's going to the bathroom.

A few minutes pass. When I do not hear water running or a toilet flushing, I think that maybe he's gone to the kitchen. A midnight snack. Yes, that must be it.

Suddenly, from down the hall, I hear a scream.

Oh, my God, I think. *Anita. Oh, my God.*

I spring off the bed, wrapping my robe around me, and dash down the hall. Anita's door is ajar. Things seem to slow down, time seems to jerk forward in a series of vignettes. I push open the door. In the light from the street lamp outside her window, I see Anita huddled in her bed, the covers pulled to her neck. Hank stands over her, wearing just his T-shirt. His pants are around his ankles. His naked ass is facing me.

"Hank! No!"

Ignoring me, Hank reaches toward Anita and yanks the covers off of her. She is wearing a T-shirt, panties. Her breasts jiggle as she pulls her knees to her chest, squishing herself against her headboard. Her eyes are wide with terror.

"Hank!" I reach out for his arm. Without looking at me, as if he were swatting away a fly, he sweeps my hand away.

"Help!" Anita is screaming now. "Help me!"

"Shut up, bitch," Hank growls. "You know you want this."

I move toward him, them, knowing that there is nothing I can do. In hand-to-hand combat, Hank can overpower both of us. All at once, as if a spring has been released inside her, Anita lunges for the nightstand by her bed. Her hand closes over something, a small canister. Her pepper spray. But she fumbles, can't get the top unscrewed. Her hand is shaking too badly.

Hank's meaty hand closes over hers. As he wrenches the canister from her hand, Anita yelps in pain.

"Fucking cunt," he snarls. "You're going to fuckin' Mace me."

He throws the pepper spray onto the floor. Then, bringing his hand back, Hank smacks her, hard, across the mouth.

Time stops.

Hank turns to me, a smile spread across his face. "You liking this, baby?" he says.

"Don't move."

We turn, all of us at once, to where Karen is standing in the doorway. She is wearing her plaid pajamas, holding a steak knife. She holds it with both hands. The little blade looks skinny and ineffectual in her hand. The light catches its silvery surface, like in a movie. Vaguely, I am aware of Hillary, the other roommate, standing just behind Karen. Her hands are at her mouth.

Anita's eyes are huge; a small, shiny drop of blood pools on her lower lip and drips onto her T-shirt, then another. A whimper escapes her lips, like a wounded animal.

I am frozen. As Hank turns to face me, I am sure he is going to attack me next. But the look on his face, incredulous, slightly amused, seems to say, *What?* His penis, still erect, gives an involuntary bob, as if doubt has spread all the way to his genitals. He looks at me, at Karen, at the knife. He pauses, an actor in a scene gauging his next move, remembering his mark.

"Oh, fuck it." He laughs, then shrugs. The scene has been played out. He can see that. To take it further is to risk parody, to cross the line from "drama" to a much more severe rating. "Bunch of silly bitches. Who needs it?" Jerking his head toward Anita, "She's a fat fucking cow, anyway." Then, as nonchalantly as if he were alone in a locker room, he hoists up his pants, zips, turns around, says, "Excuse me, ladies," and goes out the door.

No one moves. The street lamp spills just enough into the room that I can see all three of them looking at me.

A sob escapes Anita's lips. We all turn to her.

"Oh, God, Anita." I fall to my knees on the floor by her bed. "Are you all right? Oh, God, your lip." Already it's swelling, purplish blood visible beneath the skin.

"I'm calling the police," Karen says.

"No." Anita's voice is steely. "Don't bother. Just get *her* out of here."

I feel myself expand, then shrink under her glare.

"Anita, please," I say. "Let me help. I'm so sorry. I'll get you some ice . . ."

"Get *out*." Anita's voice has an hysterical edge to it now.

Numbly, I turn and go down the hall to my room. The door is open. Hank and his clothes are gone. I sit down on my bed. My mind moves forward haltingly, like an engine that won't catch.

I must do something.

I go into the kitchen, wrap ice cubes in a paper towel, head back to Anita's room.

Karen and Hillary are gathered around her bed. Hillary is stroking her hair. Karen is speaking softly.

"Here." I hold out the ice pack to Anita, a pathetic favor. The other girls move closer to Anita, protectively, closing the space around her.

My hands are shaking, so that the ice cubes rattle like teeth chattering.

Carefully, as if it might be poisoned, Karen takes the ice pack. She hands it to Anita, who holds it to her lip. They all look at me, with a cold levelness in their eyes that makes my heart freeze. Their eyes say, *Get out.*

And I do.

Somehow, the night passes. I lay rigid on my bed, in the grip of a familiar, pounding terror, the terror I feel thinking about the surgery compounded by the horror of what happened last night. Night drains from the sky; the first streaks of dawn appear like rents in a dark fabric. I hear voices, the girls talking softly down the hall. It seems they have not slept, either. I go down the hall. They are sitting on Anita's bed. She has put on a sweatshirt and sweatpants. Her lip, when she takes the ice pack away, is huge. When I appear, the conversation stops.

"I . . ." What can I say? "I'm so sorry. I didn't know this was going to happen."

The girls look at each other. Then, as if on cue, Karen speaks. It appears this has been rehearsed among them.

"Look, Hope. You have to move out. If you move out as soon as possible, we won't call the police on your friend. Okay?"

The words register with a dull shock. *Move out. Police. Your friend.* Friend? Hank is not my friend. A friend is someone you like, someone you have something in common with. Hank is just . . . what is he? He is nothing.

Karen keeps talking. Her voice is controlled, firm, but I hear a tremor in it. I keep wanting to glance behind me, to see who it is they are talking to. *You don't understand!* I want to shout. *This isn't really me. It's just an experiment I'm doing! I'm only pretending to be someone else. I don't know who I am, don't you see, I have no idea, I'm lost, and if I can't figure out who I am then maybe I can define myself by who I'm not! I'm not this careless, out of control person you see in front of you, I don't want to be her. Just give me a chance. Don't make me leave!* I want to beg, to cry. I feel the sting of tears behind my eyes. Maybe I can make them understand, I think. Maybe if I throw myself on their mercy, if I beg forgiveness . . .

"I think you'll agree this is not working out," Karen continues, speaking evenly. It strikes me then: She is afraid of me. They are all afraid of me. "You eat our food. You take our things. Do you think we don't notice? We should have said something to you a long time ago."

"Why didn't you?" I ask, feeling suddenly, terribly sorry. How could I have been so oblivious, so thoughtless?

"We should have. We know that. But it's just that we felt sorry for you."

Sorry for me? Her words are a slap in the face. Something hardens inside me. A door slams shut. I force the tears back. I look at the three of them and think, *You are my enemies now. My opponents.* I won't let them see me cry. I won't show any weakness. Sorry. They feel sorry for me. I'll make them sorry.

My hands are shaking. Even through my anger, it occurs to me that if I stay calm, if I reiterate my apology, I may not change their minds but I will, at least, retrieve some of my self-respect. I will have done the right thing. But another part of me feels small and mean and desperate.

"*Fuck* you," I snarl.

I turn slowly and stroll down the hall to my room, adding a colossal slam of my door that rattles the apartment. This, I think, is something they'd expect of me.

I sit on my bed, shaken and horrified. What has just happened? What have I done? That sneering stranger, that animal backed into a corner baring its teeth—that is not me. I'm a good girl. I'm a Hathaway. This is not me. And yet, I can't go back now. I can't undo what I've done. There is something liberating about my bad behavior, something welcome and refreshing in the force of my rage. I feel as if I've tapped at last into a part of myself I've kept hidden all these years. Now—in a glorious burst of *so-the-fuck-what!*—I am letting loose. It feels giddy, strange, powerful. Almost transporting. I feel like Godzilla, looking around at all the tiny, shrieking people. I want to destroy something.

Over the next few hours, unable to sleep, I feel myself go into a kind of survival mode. Everything I think and feel becomes stream-lined, until I don't feel anything at all. I lie on the bed, feeling a dull knocking in my chest. I have to remind myself it is my heart.

Down the hall, I hear the girls begin the motions of their day. I listen, an outsider now, an unwanted stranger, as their lives carry on as usual. They had a problem, me, and now that problem is solved. It is business as usual.

My life, however, has stopped.

All day, I lie on the bed, staring at a single hairline crack in the blank white ceiling. I do not flinch, shift, or go to the bathroom. I have never lain so long in one position, without moving, even after a surgery. I think, idly, that perhaps I have become paralyzed, suf-fered a stroke and am now immobile. When the breeze coming through my window lifts a lock of my hair, I startle.

Sometime in the late afternoon, my eyes scratchy and stinging, my anger returns, the same anger I felt the previous night, only stronger, more specific and definable. I feel my mind narrow itself into a long, thin tube like the barrel of a gun. At the end of that barrel, squarely in my sight, is Hank.

Hank. It is suddenly, shockingly clear to me that my entire situation is his fault. He is the reason all this has happened to me. In spite of my rage, it is a profound relief to know this, like applying a cool compress to a burn. *He* is responsible for my misery. *He* has caused me to lose something of utmost importance, my living accommodations. My self-respect, too. I am nothing more than a blow-up doll to him. Therefore, he must pay. He must be forced to lose something similarly important of his. The thought has a satisfying logic.

I spring from my bed, feeling energized despite my lack of sleep, and begin to form a P-L-A-N.

I've already figured out, of course, that Hank probably had some wife or girlfriend at home. I will find out where they live. I'll expose him for the cheating, lying, sex-crazed bastard he is. I'll ruin his life! The details are fuzzy, but the idea of revenge makes me feel much, much better. Brilliant, strong, full of purpose. Brave. Almost whole again.

But first things first. It is near the end of the month. I will be able to find another apartment. My lease is month-to-month. It won't be hard. There are FOR RENT signs all over the neighborhood. But I can't move until after I've recovered from the surgery, at least a little. I write my roommates a curt note.

Don't worry, I will be moving out shortly. You can
expect that I will be gone by the end of April. I
hope that you will give me this much time to
arrange a new domicile. I would most appreciate it.
Thank you.
With Best Regards,
Hope

Reading it over again, the brittle frailty and stiff defensiveness makes me want to cry. *Karen will probably feel even more sorry for me when she reads this,* I think, slipping it under her door.

Next, I dig under my bed for Hank's headshot. He had given it to me a few weeks ago, a lapse in his otherwise vigilant reticence about his personal life. It is so typically Hank, I think now: He does not want me to know the first thing about him, yet he cannot resist handing out a glossy picture of himself.

I turn it over, figuring it must have some contact information. Bingo! There is a phone number. No address, but a phone number. Okay. Now what? Think.

My mind is working very quickly and efficiently, better than it has in months. I look at the clock: 6:00 p.m. Most likely, Hank is already at the theater getting ready for the play. Before I can change my mind, I pick up the phone and dial.

A girl answers.

"Is Hank there?" I say.

"He's not home right now," says the girl. "Can I give him a message?" She sounds young, fresh, unsuspecting. I hear water running in the background and picture her standing over a kitchen sink, washing Hank's dirty dishes.

"Is this his girlfriend?" I ask cheerily.

"Yes."

Ah-ha! Bastard! I charge ahead. "I'm a friend of his from the play," I say, keeping my voice light and casual. "A while ago, he lent me some of your videotapes, and I've been meaning to return them for so long, and I just haven't. I'm so sorry." It shocks me how convincing and unaffected I sound.

"Oh, that's okay!" chirps the girl. "Don't worry about it."

"Anyway, I'm going to be in the area tomorrow morning, very early, and I thought I'd just drop them in your mailbox, if that's all right."

"Sure!" says the girl.

"Can you tell me your address?"

I feel a little guilty, she is so nice. She sounds so . . . *clueless* is the only word that comes to mind. Poor thing. How can such a nice girl be Hank's girlfriend?

When we hang up, I get in my car and drive west on the 10 to Venice. The house, a ramshackle beach bungalow, is easy to find.

I park across the street. Some of my conviction wavers, but I tell myself it's just fatigue catching up with me. So this is Hank's house, I think. It is, now that I'm staring at it, rather disappointing. Depressing, actually. Is this how struggling actors live? A single bare bulb dangling over the front door, a few leggy rosebushes lining the path to the front door, starbursts of dried crabgrass pushing through the cracked concrete.

I realize that I have no idea what I plan to do, now that I am here.

I run through my options. Go up and ring the doorbell and run away? That would be silly. Wait for the girl to answer and angrily confront her? *I'm your rival,* I might say. Suddenly, it doesn't seem worth the effort. It seems absurd. All the wind goes out of my sails. What the hell am I doing here?

I feel a dark, heavy depression begin to settle over me. All this planning and scheming . . . for what? For someone whom I didn't even give a shit about? My anger, the rush of victory I felt, fade to nothing. The wasted effort of it, the sheer hopelessness, makes me want to cry. Aren't I, I think pathetically, aren't I *better* than this? Shouldn't I be *above* such nonsense?

Abruptly, overwhelmingly tired, I contemplate taking a nap in my car. The dead weight of fatigue presses behind my eyeballs, making them ache.

I am about to close my eyes when, ten feet away from me, across the street, Hank's car pulls into the driveway. The familiar outline of his big head is framed in the streetlight.

I freeze, squishing myself down in my seat so that my eyes are level with the steering wheel.

Oh, shit.

Hank will be furious to know I've tracked him down. What will he do? If he struck Anita for nothing, what would he do to me?

My brain clicks quickly through the facts: I will be moving in a few weeks. I won't tell him where I'm going. But for now, he knows where I live. He can easily come after me. Who knew if I could resist his blows any more energetically than I'd resisted his advances? Will I become the same hapless rag doll during a fight as I was during sex?

Desperately, I will him not to look across the street. As for my car, I think: There are thousands of red Jeeps in L.A., right?

Hank has parked the car and switched off the lights. I can't see what he's doing, but it appears he is gathering something from the passenger seat.

Please don't look over here, I silently beseech him. *Please, please don't see me.*

But the man who gets out of the car a moment later doesn't look at all like Hank. He is stooped, for one thing, his shoulders rounded over in a discouraged-looking posture. Instead of looking tall and strong, he looks defeated. In place of the usual tight black T-shirt, he wears a faded button-down of some lumpy, unattractive plaid.

Hank? I think. *Hank, is that you?*

As he ambles up to the front door, he raises his hand to scratch the back of his neck. The light from the bare bulb catches his familiar gold ring with the bucking horse on it.

Stunned, I think: So he *does* change in the car! I am in shock. The man walking up to the house does not look like a leading man, or someone who would be in a movie with Dolph Lundgren. He looks like a plumber, weary and resigned, coming home from a long day of snaking clogged drains. He looks like someone who would be named Hank.

The door opens, and a girl steps out to greet him. She is drying her hands on a dishcloth as he reaches out and pecks her on the cheek. She is talking animatedly to him, her mouth moving, smiling. I stare hard at her, looking for a clue as to who Hank really is. She has bleached-blonde hair with the dark roots grown out a little, not fashionably so, but as if she dyes it herself and simply hasn't gotten around to it lately.

They go inside, and the door closes behind them. The bulb swings listlessly.

So this is the real Hank, I think. Maybe he isn't an actor after all. Maybe the only acting he does is at different women's houses, like mine, performing for an indifferent audience of one.

I almost feel sorry for him. What does he do to support himself and the girl, whoever she is? She had seemed so happy to see him, chattering away. Telling him, I imagined, about her day.

All down the block, lights are coming on in the shabby houses. I start my car and just sit there. I don't know where to go.

I do not feel jealous watching Hank and the girl. I don't feel anything at all. How could I mistake this lack of feeling, this numbness, for victory? With the almost-hunger pangs I feel earlier pulling at my insides, I am acutely aware of how empty my stomach is, how empty I am. I am so tired. Too tired to drive, too tired to do anything at all but sit in my car on this unfamiliar street, where a bustle of evening activity has begun. Men and women are coming home from work, children are being called in for dinner. I have had this feeling my whole life, the feeling that life is something that happens to other people. It's as if I've accidentally stepped off the escalator of life and am watching, forlorn and helpless, while everyone else passes by. I wish that the emptiness inside me could be more specific; an answerable need, even an actual physical pain. Any of those things, anything, would be easier to alleviate than the dull ache of longing inside me, the drowning pull of depression. There. I have said it: depression. I am deeply, profoundly depressed. Why does it feel like such a failure to admit this?

I watch the shapes of Hank and the girl moving back and forth behind a tattered curtain in what looks like a dining room, perhaps setting a table. *I wouldn't be caught dead living in a house like that,* a little voice in my mind snaps, a bitter, defensive voice, my mother's voice. A television is switched on, the eerie flickering blue-green light like an alien spaceship. I think of something I read about people who claim to have been abducted by aliens in their sleep. They were, almost as a rule, single people, lonely, bereft, though they would be the last ones to admit this. It was their own deeply denied loneliness which triggered a belief that alien visitors had singled them out for visitation, examination, sometimes even artificial insemination. They sometimes felt "violated." Unable to admit their own yearning for intimacy, they conjured alien beings who touched them in ways they were not touched in everyday life.

Sitting in my car, now, I understand this. I feel very acutely how this could be so. When you are in enough pain, you will settle for anything that promises even a smidgen of comfort, no matter how bizarre. The more bizarre, the better, because it is too vast, too huge and scary, to admit that you want Love, and Purpose, and A Life. I *want,* and the wanting feels so huge and overwhelming that I must try to narrow it to a specific need. Higher cheekbones. Bigger breasts. Dr. S—'s fickle attention. Hank's empty desire. All these "solutions" are as ephemeral as smoke, each thrill as brief as a sugar rush.

Sitting in my aimlessly idling car outside of Hank's house I feel, I think, exactly what those people visited by aliens must feel upon waking: alone. Briefly visited, momentarily moved, but alone. Again.

CHAPTER 21

There is a truck parked on my chest. Shallow, halting breaths are all I can bear to take. I can't turn or breathe deeply or cry. I don't want to move from my bed. Once the morphine wears off, knives stab viciously at my chest. Rolling over is out of the question. Going to the bathroom is an ordeal; the exertion of getting up and taking a few steps makes me pant and weep with agony.

It is April Fools' Day, and I have new breasts.

I lie on my back, trying not to breathe, trying not to move, tears leaking out of my eyes and pooling coldly in my ears. Occasionally I hear the fall of my roommates' footsteps in the hall. They do not know I had surgery; I wonder if any of them are curious as to what has happened to me. I have not been out of my room in two days. Probably they think I am just avoiding them. Still, I make extra noise on my infrequent trips to the bathroom, rustling drawers and running the water full blast, caught up in a desperate need to believe that Karen, Anita, and Hillary, somewhere on the other side of the door, will be reassured to know that I am still alive.

My mother calls. I cannot roll over to reach for the phone, so I listen to her chirpy voice coming out of the answering machine. She and my father have found a house in Pasadena, they'll move in two months, it's a wonderful Ranch-style home with a kidney-shaped pool. "And you'll have to choose which room you want," she says. "There is one I think you'll love that looks out on the pool."

When she hangs up I want to weep. I stare at the little red blinking light on the answering machine as if it is my only link to real life.

A sudden, intense, red-hot burning below my left armpit makes me gasp. My flesh is on fire from within. I am being seared. I want to scream. This must be the sensation Dr. S— warned me about, the muscle rubbing against the implant, around which my body has not yet formed a barrier of protective scar tissue. "Like a rope burn," he said, making it sound like nothing. But oh, this pain! Is this the "mild to moderate discomfort" he said I might experience?

I watch the clock by my bed, watch as each minute ticks slowly by. Is this much pain normal? I consider calling Dr. S—'s answering exchange. He is out of town for the weekend, but there is another doctor on call. I don't feel like talking to a stranger. I feel a sudden rush of anger: Dr. S— said that he usually sees his post-op breast patients two days after surgery, but because he was going away, he wouldn't be able to see me for five. I would be, he assured me, perfectly all right.

I try, now, to focus on my breathing, taking the sort of quick, shallow breaths women in labor take. I manage to spill two little white pain pills into my hand, gulp them down dry.

I fall asleep with tears drying on my cheeks, leaving stiff, salty trails I can taste with my tongue.

The following Monday morning, I wince as Dr. S— slides the tight surgical bra off my shoulders.

"These are looking *very* nice." Dr. S—'s voice is husky. "Oh, yes. Very nice. Are you having any discomfort?"

Discomfort? I think, incredulous. Is this something they teach doctors to say in medical school? In addition to the constant, stabbing pain, there is the burning sensation, and a flu-like ache in my entire body. When I tell him this, fearing I might have an infection, Dr. S— reassures me that it is all normal. I have been cut into, after all, the muscles and tissue are being stretched out, and my body is reacting to what it knows are two foreign objects inside it. After a week or so, he says, when it realizes it cannot expel them, my body will start forming scar tissue around each implant, surrounding the potentially dangerous intruders within stiff little capsules.

I look down at my breasts. They are feverishly hot to the touch, and there is a line of black stitches tracing the red smile of the incision beneath each nipple. There is also, above my left aureole, a distinct thumb-shaped bruise, as if he'd had to jam the implant in with an unusual force. I can, I think, almost make out Dr. S—'s fingerprint.

"You must be very happy with these," he says, in a husky voice which tells me that he himself is very happy with them, and leaves no room for the possibility that I might not be.

"I'll be happier when the pain goes away, but, um, I'm h-h-happy." The word comes out as a stutter, a lie that won't quite trip off my tongue. Still, I want him to be proud of me. Just the effort of talking is excruciating. Driving here, I thought I would pass out from the pain. In fact, Dr. S— had told me not to drive a car for at least a week afterward. But who else do I have to drive me?

"Good, Hope. I'm glad to hear it. That's the way we like it."

There is a soft rap on the door, followed by Alana's soft, deferential voice. "Mrs. Shultz is here," she says.

"Right there!" he calls. Then, to me: "So I'll see you in a week, Hope. We'll get those stitches out, and then, basically, you're on auto-pilot." He turns and heads for the door.

"Doctor!" That word. It still thrills me, a thrill that cuts through the pain. I am breathless, but it could be the dressings, the constricting after-surgery bra. *Please stay here and talk to me some more,* I want to beg. *Please don't leave me to go back to my apartment and be all alone again, so soon. Please don't call my pain discomfort.*

"Is there anything special I should or shouldn't do?" I ask.

"Anything you should or shouldn't do, huh? Hm. Let me think." Dr. S— looks thoughtful as he turns my question over in his mind. "There is one thing," he says.

"Yes?" It takes all my effort not to cry. "What is it?"

"Don't let anyone put their lips on them for a week." With a playful wink, Dr. S— closes the door and is gone.

CHAPTER 22

I am nearly broke. I need money. I tell myself that this is why I answer the ad, in the classified section of a local newspaper, one of those throwaway weeklies stacked high at coffee shops and bookstores. The ad says, in bold capital letters: FIGURE MODELS WANTED, NO EXPERIENCE, FAST $$$.

I've moved into a tiny, dingy studio apartment off of King's Road in West Hollywood. The carpet smells of cat piss, but I was so grateful that they didn't bother to check my credit, I signed the lease immediately.

I keep the little ad for a week or so before answering it. I like the sound of it: Figure Modeling. It has a nice, artsy ring to it. Like something out of Degas. Figure modeling. It sounds so quaint, so old-fashioned. Of course, a part of me knows that it isn't going to be this innocent. Especially when the ad is placed alongside those advertising escort services, sensual massage, and phone-sex lines. I know I will not be posing chastely for a master drawing class. I know, too, that the reason I am answering the ad is not entirely because I am broke.

It has come down to this: I have only my body and face to offer. I am so caught up in my physical self that I believe it is all I have to offer, all that I am. Even my needs and intentions feel naked, stripped of illusion; I cannot fool myself anymore that I am improving my life, that I am on a path to something significant, that Dr. S— will love me. There is, I feel, only day-to-day survival, the next fleeting thrill. I want someone to save me, even temporarily, and to this end I will lay bare not just my body but also my soul, offer anything and everything. There is a kind of honesty to my desperation, a spiritual quality. My degradation feels, at times, almost divine, a sort of martyrdom. But for whom am I martyring myself? What good is subjugation, without someone to subjugate myself to? I have nothing but myself to offer, nothing more to lose. Naked, I will ask for love, for approval, for attention. I will implore, cajole, seduce.

I find the address the man on the phone gives, the second floor of a run-down office building in the Valley, across from a Ralph's supermarket, sandwiched between Bev's Beauty Temple and Le Sex Shoppe. I wonder, vaguely, in which order a person might visit these establishments: first the Temple and then the Shoppe, or the Shoppe and then the Temple?

I follow the signs up a dingy flight of stairs through an open door to a darkish room with no windows. A man stands up from behind a desk. He extends his hand to me, but I cannot quite make out his face.

"You must be Faith," he says. "Frank North."

"It's Hope," I correct him, sounding, I think, uncharacteristically prim. "How do you do."

North's hand is thin and papery, giving way when I take it with a small cracking sound, like chicken bones crunching. The room smells, predictably, of stale cigarette smoke.

"Have a seat, Hope," he says, indicating a chair in front of his desk whose sagging vinyl cushion gives way with an unflattering rush of air. "My mistake. Let's see, Faith, Hope, and Charity? No, that's not it. I can see you're not one of the three virtues!"

I manage a dry laugh. Now that he is seated, with the lamp on his desk illuminating him, I see what he looks like. He is not old, perhaps in his mid-fifties, but he has an aged look about him. Lots of deep wrinkles, grayish smoker's skin. Only his hair seems alert and alive, a swell of black hair combed up and back into a pompadour. He does not seem like a pervert, or an ax murderer.

I relax a little.

"So, Hope, you said on the phone you'd done some modeling before."

"I've never done any *nude* modeling."

"Ah. Well, any experience in front of a camera helps, eh? What kind of modeling did you do, dear?"

I'm looking around the room at the glossy framed photos of pretty women in different poses and stages of undress, hefting various overlarge body parts into the camera lens like ripe, flushed fruit. At the other end of the narrow room, another, younger man is talking on a telephone. "I did a hair ad once, in high school," I say. "For a local salon. It ran in the newspaper."

"Which newspaper?"

"The *Larchmont Chronicle*."

"Can't say as I've heard of it."

"It's a small paper. In Hancock Park."

"Hancock Park?" North's eyebrows bob up, then down. "Isn't that where all the rich people live?"

"Yeah, well . . ."

Before I can finish, North is calling to the man across the room.

"Hey, Tom!" he says. "This here young lady is from Hancock Park!"

Tom puts his hand over the receiver and says, "Ooh la-la."

Maybe I should have said Iowa or Kansas or something, I think. But that would just make me seem poor and hokey and desperate, instead of . . . instead of what? Rich and sophisticated and desperate? Well-bred and intelligent and desperate? No matter what else I am, that adjective remains firmly attached.

I clear my throat.

I am wearing the long, streaky blonde wig today, fearing that my own short hair is not sexy enough. I struggled with the wig for a long time this morning, sweating and swearing, trying to position it so that it looked natural. Never having worn a wig before, I was surprised at how difficult it is. I secured it, finally, with bobby pins, pulling out a few wisps of my own hair to make it look, if not natural, at least all right. It feels like a dead animal on my head.

From inside his desk North produces a clipboard with some papers on it and hands it to me.

"Here's a list of the kinds of work our girls do and the money they make," he says. "Also a few forms we need you to fill out."

Girls? I think. Shouldn't girls who take their clothes off for money at least be given the more respectful, adult title of women? This is, I remind myself, not the time to be a feminist. A latent Gloria Steinem tendency, if indeed I have one, will not be met with applause in this office.

I take the papers and look them over, my eyes skimming immediately to the bottom of the page, where the largest amounts of money are. "What do you mean by multiples?" I ask, though this seems obvious.

"That means you're with more than one partner," North says. "Of course, that's films we're talking about."

"Good Lord!" I say, then immediately regret it. Good *Lord?* Why did my mother's expressions come to me, at a time like this? I adjust my purse strap back onto my shoulder and cross my legs, smoothing down the hem of my short blue batik-print sundress, trying not to appear rattled. "I just mean, God. I'm not interested in doing any porno films."

"Of course not," North says. "I understand completely."

"And interracial?" I ask, though this, too, must be self-explanatory.

"Films, again," North says. "Some ladies don't like to be with a black guy."

"Really?" I say. "It seems sort of silly that someone who's going to have sex with a stranger on film would object to that person's skin color, don't you think? I mean, wouldn't that be the *last* of your worries?"

North tips back in his chair, taps his fingers together, smiles at me. "I like this girl," he says to Tom across the room, who has hung up the phone and is now following our conversation. To me he says, "I like how you think, young lady. You're a spirited little filly."

I think of my favorite book as a child, *Misty of Chincoteague*. A spirited filly, huh? I'd give him spirited. "Don't worry, I'm not going to ask you what 'anal' means," I say.

"Well that's a relief," he says. "I don't go in much for having to explain the birds and the bees to people."

North, I am certain, has a sense of himself as something of a character, and does what he can to exaggerate it. Tom makes his way across the room and sits on a couch against the wall, next to North and me. They are both looking at me with an interested, slightly bemused expression that seems to say, *What have we here?*

I feel myself grow warm under their attention. My shoulders relax. I consider telling them I was a debutante, knowing this would really make an impression. How many former debutantes have walked through these doors? It could be my claim to fame, the thing that sets me apart. Good girl gone bad, poor little rich girl. I'm trying on personas again, but this time, I think I may be on to something. I feel, here in this office, with North and Tom, more at ease than I've felt in months. Is it possible that, in this most unlikely of settings, I may have found myself? Could I possibly be a porno star, appalling as it sounds?

"I guess I should, you know, make it clear right now that there are certain things I *won't* do," I say, realizing, as I say it, that I am not sure exactly what those things are. How many things have I done in the past months that I never thought I'd do? What *wouldn't* I do?

"Before we go any further," North says, stubbing out his cigarette, "I need to have a look at your driver's license."

"My driver's license? What do you need that for?"

"Just procedure," says North. "Something we ask everyone. We need to be sure of your age, is all. Had a little fiasco with a girl named Traci Lords a few years back. Do you know who Traci Lords is?"

"Of course I know who Traci Lords is." I feel slightly insulted. "Do I look that prudish? I'm from L.A., not rat-fuck Kansas."

"'Course." North chuckles. "We had some trouble, what with Traci being underage and all," he says. "Can't afford to have that ol' laissez-faire attitude about age no more after that." The way he says it sounds like "Lassie fair."

I fumble in my purse for my license, reaching it across the desk to him. A thin veil of sweat prickles my forehead, under my bangs, but I am afraid to wipe it away for fear my wig will go askew.

"I know you're interested in being a figure model," North says, glancing at my license before putting it on the desk in front of him, satisfied. "That's all fine and good. But why don't we talk about some options." He folds his hands on his desk, leaning forward in what I assume is his "let's talk business" pose.

I study him. He has a strange sort of saggy face. It isn't enough to say that he simply has wrinkles. Rather, the skin hangs loosely on the bones in such a way that it appears as if he is melting. Heavy smoking has made his skin look waxy and artificial, almost as if it stretches uneasily over the bones, cringing a little.

"Most of our girls start in modeling," he says. "Or dancing. We have *a lot* of exotic dancers." He makes this sound like something special, something worth boasting about, making me think of the representatives from Ivy League colleges who came to my high school during junior year, saying, "*Thirty percent* of our graduates become doctors or lawyers!"

"Everyone says they won't do films at first," North continues.

"But films," he shakes his head, casting his eyes heavenward as if this is something which can't be helped. "Films are where the money is." His black hair is the same color as his vinyl chair, I notice, and as shiny. "Tom here was the same way"— he nods at Tom, who bobs his head in a kind of resigned agreement—"and now he's one of my top performers. Isn't that right, Tom?"

"True," says Tom, obviously a man of few words. I look at Tom, study him. I can't hide my surprise. He does not look like an adult film star. A tight, white T-shirt pulls at his beefy arms. His neck is thick and blockish. He isn't terribly handsome, or sexy, just average. I imagine he must have a similarly thick, stocky penis, the blue-collar worker of penises. "You're a . . ."—what had North called him?—"a performer?"

"Yes, ma'am," he says.

"Wow," I say. "I wouldn't have known."

"Yep, we're just everyday people," North says, and I instantly regret having given him such an easy segue into this remark. "Just everyday working people."

Looking at Tom, I think, for an instant, of what it would be like to have sex with him. It doesn't excite or arouse me. The term "getting down to business" comes to mind. But it doesn't seem impossible. I'm ashamed by how quickly my mind veers in that direction. But, I think, it really isn't much different than meeting a guy at a party—Hank, for example—and sizing him up, is it? It doesn't mean anything.

Feeling a bit disconcerted, I try to steer the conversation back to modeling. "How much money are we talking about, just for basic nude pictures? Not films, just photos. Say, *Playboy.*"

Tom and North look at each other, exchange sort of indulgent smiles.

"Well, let me tell you now, *Playboy*'s tough," North says, with the kind tone of a father telling his child, as gently as possible, that her dream might not come true. "They tend to use their own girls. I'm not saying it's impossible, but it's tough."

"Ah," I say. So much for *Playboy*. I should have known they wouldn't seek out the likes of North for their models. I feel silly and embarrassed, like a naïve wannabe actress who's announced that she wants to be Julia Roberts.

"Tell you what." North stands up. "Before we go any further, let's take a few Polaroids."

I follow him into a smaller, adjoining room, thinking, *Here we go. You knew this was coming. Don't pretend you didn't.*

North closes the door behind us.

"Take off your clothes," he says, pulling a ratty shade down over the single small window. "Don't worry, I'm just like a doctor. Seen thousands of bodies."

For a moment I think of the stacks of *Playboy* magazines in my grandfather's study, of my mother quipping, "You'd think he'd seen enough of *that* at the hospital all day, wouldn't you?" I picture North in a white doctor's coat, a speculum in his hand. The thought makes me want to laugh.

I hesitate, knowing there is something I have to tell him.

"I have scars on my breasts," I say. "From having implants put in. They're not too bad, but they're still noticeable."

"Don't worry about that," North says. "Most of our girls have those. Let's have a look."

"All right."

With trembling hands, I undo the buttons of my dress and let the thin fabric slide off my shoulders. The dress lands in a neat circle around my feet, like a lasso. I step out of it. North is fussing with the Polaroid camera, putting in some film. I reach around and undo my bra, then slide my panties down my legs. I toss them both on top of the dress.

North looks up. "Sweet *Je*-sus," he says. "Will you marry me?"

I know, suddenly and fully, why I am here. This reaction, this attention, this desire. However fleeting, however insincere. I smile, feeling my cheeks flush.

"You must say that to everyone," I say.

"Believe me, I don't," he says.

I want to believe him.

North stares at my breasts. "Those scars aren't too bad. When did you have the implants put in?"

"A little over a month ago."

"Oh. Well, hell, that's why they're still red. Do you have a lip pencil or something?"

"I think so." I reach in my purse, take out my nude-colored lip liner. "Do you want me to color them in?" I ask.

He nods.

While North watches, I cup one breast and then the other, tracing the outline of each aureole with the lip pencil, then blending the color around my nipples.

"Perfect. Now just relax. Be yourself."

Relax? I think. *Be myself?* Those are two things I do not know how to do.

North moves in a circle around me. "Put your hand on your hip," he says. "That's good. Nice. Lean your upper body forward just a little." The camera clicks, spitting out pictures which North holds in his other hand.

I am having trouble thinking of places to put my hands. I feel a little awkward and self-conscious, as if no matter what I do, I end up in a sort of coy beauty queen pose, with one leg slightly bent at the knee, hips squared, a serene smile on my face.

"What do you do with the pictures?" I ask.

North has finished the roll, and is pulling the last one through the camera.

"We put them in a book." Suddenly, it seems he's turned brisk and businesslike. No nonsense. "See you back in the office." He doesn't wait for me to dress, but is already out the door, which he leaves open, waving the developing Polaroids in his hand like a fan.

A book? I think. What kind of book? A book anyone can look at? I hurry after him, buttoning the last buttons of my dress. "Can, um, anybody look at them?"

"Not anybody," North says. "That's how the producers and photographers find you."

I have a feeling of being duped. Producers? Didn't I just say I wouldn't consider doing films?

North spreads the Polaroids out on his desk. Tom leans over his shoulder and they study them together, nodding. I watch North select one, put it on the desk beside my driver's license, and copy my name, my real, full name, in black felt-tip marker under the photograph.

Tom says, "You might think about a stage name."

"Don't pressure the girl," North says, before I can answer. "Give her a chance."

From inside his desk, North pulls out a thick, leather-bound photo album, the kind that might be filled with family photographs. He opens it at random and I can see that it is full of Polaroids like mine. As he flips through the plastic sleeves, I catch glimpses of naked skin, pale and overexposed in the camera's flash, shadows of pubic hair, dark dots of nipples. There must be hundreds of women in the album. I blink in disbelief.

After flipping a few pages, North finds an empty slot, slips my picture inside, and snaps the album shut.

My heart is beating so hard I think it will punch out my throat.

"Don't look so nervous," North says. "It's not like we're going to force you to do anything."

"No one back in Hancock Park is going to see this," says Tom.

I manage a weak smile.

"You're a beautiful girl," North says. "You'll get a lot of work. It's up to you to decide what you want to do. *You* call the shots." He leans across the desk so that his melting face is just inches from mine. "Let me tell you something," he says. His breath is surprisingly odorless, for someone who smokes and who looks so aggressively unhealthy. "What we do, here in this business, is no different than a girl who goes out on a Friday night, meets a guy, and has herself a big time. People like to think it's different, get all high and mighty about it, but it's not. What we're putting on film is the same thing people are doing in their apartments. If you ask me, it's more honest. Everyone fucks, right? Everyone gets off. It's no different. Is it, Tom?"

"No different," says Tom.

"I see your point," I say. "You make a very good case." I realize, then, that I have come to a point when I can either walk out, or stay.

"Look, why don't we talk about this more over lunch," North says. "My blood sugar's low. When you get to be my age, you have to worry about things like that." He winks at me, fatherly. "You'll join us, won't you, Hope?"

I look from North to Tom, at both of the men's mild, expectant faces. I want the feeling I had a few minutes ago, light, a little bit high on their attention, lifted out of myself.

"C'mon, Gorgeous," North says. "Let us buy you lunch."

I don't have to tell them that I'm not going to make movies, I think. I can just string them along a little.

"Why not?" I hear myself say. "I'd love to."

I look up at North and find that he is already ushering me out the door, with just the slightest insistent pressure of his hand on my elbow, as if he had doubted only for a moment what my answer would be.

"Shall we, my dear?" he says.

We eat at a deli across the street. North selects a table outside, on a patio in the sun. I pull the dress down a little, exposing my shoulders, soaking up the warmth.

There are people at tables all around us, normal, everyday working people, and we do not look any different. Two men join us, whom North introduces as a film producer and a grip, and we sit, the five of us, in the midst of this normalness. I have a Cobb salad and a Coke. North orders beers, which I decline. The grip sits to my right. He is a quiet, heavyset young man in his early twenties. I am not sure exactly what a grip does, but I gather it is something to do with lights. He keeps sneaking glances at me, in a way that is oddly bashful for someone who lights naked bodies all day.

After a while, I realize that I am completely relaxed, at ease with them. There is something in their easy camaraderie that feels lulling, comfortable. I like being here with them. I do not want our lunch to end. I feel popular, flirty, the new girl in high school whom everyone wants to get to know. The producer seems so benign that I don't even flinch when North says to him casually, halfway through lunch, "Why don't you come back to the office and see Hope's Polaroids?"

"I'd like to, but I can't," he replies. "I've got to pick my kids up at school. It's my day to get them."

He has to pick up his kids at school, I think. *How much more normal can you get?* "What does your wife do?" I ask politely.

"She used to be in the business," he says, sort of muttering, so that I have to strain to hear him.

"You mean"— what was the word North had used?—"as an actress?"

"A performer," corrects North, through a mouthful of turkey sandwich.

"Not anymore, though," the producer says quickly, and I wonder if I am imagining the slight shameful edge to his voice.

"Hope is from Hancock Park," North says. "You know, where all the old mansions are?"

The men murmur admiringly.

"So what are you doing here?" one of them says.

"I, um . . . I need to—"

"That's exactly the question *I* asked her," North says, forgetting that he had not asked me this. "You sure you're not some rich girl slummin' it, seeing how the other half lives?" The men laugh. "You're not some fuckin' debutante just tryin' to piss off her parents, are you?"

"Actually . . ." How should I play this? "I was a debutante."

"Well." North sits back in his chair. "Gentlemen, we are in the presence of royalty. Ah, c'mon, Hope, don't go getting all pouty on me. We're just teasin'."

"I know," I shrug, to show I don't care. And the funny thing is, I don't. I'm acting. I feel like I'm in a scene in a movie. "I can take it."

"You've gotta have a thick skin in this business," North says. Then, turning to the men: "Hope was asking about films. We told her that's where the money is."

"What do you do now?" Tom asks me.

"I'm an actress." The lie slips out of my mouth so easily it startles me. "An aspiring actress," I add quickly, in case they might ask what roles I've had. "But I'm temping now, to pay my rent."

"Better money than that," says North, lighting a cigarette. "Films are where the money is." This seems to be his mantra.

"I've got a spot on a film this week," says the producer, dabbing at his mouth with a napkin. "I need a girl for a couple of scenes."

"What kind of scenes?" I ask. "I mean, just out of curiosity."

"Not fucking," North says, smoke exiting the corners of his mouth in two neat lines, like a dragon's breath. "No screwing or nothing. Maybe a blow job. Or a girl-on-girl scene."

"Oh, no," I say quickly, holding up my palm like a stop sign. "There's no way I would—"

"Why don't we do this," North interrupts, signaling the waiter to bring our check. "You could come and just watch, Hope. See how you feel. Get comfortable around the set, if you want."

Nearby a man tucks a lettuce leaf into his mouth; a woman gives a tinkling laugh. All around us life carries on, ordinary, upbeat. It seems incredible that I am actually giving this consideration. And yet, where is the harm in it? "Just watch." How many people get an opportunity to watch a porno film being made? It would be—in my favorite father's words—a unique experience.

"I might do that," I say. "But I still want to do figure modeling. I really need to get some work right away."

"Sure, that goes without saying." North signs the check with a flourish. "You'll get lots of work. A girl like you doesn't walk in here every day. You'll be turning *down* work, let me tell you. Am I right? Gentlemen?"

The men nod, murmuring agreement.

"Oh, yeah," says one.

"She's gorgeous," says another.

My head is spinning. I look down, feeling the heat of their eyes on me. Very daintily, I pick a piece of bacon out of my salad, put it on my bread plate. Affecting the voice of a flustered Southern belle, I drawl, "Ma goodness, fellas, y'all better stop." I feel giddy, fearless, powerful. All self-consciousness has drained out of me. I am vibrating with the hum of this moment, of being wanted, of being *seen*.

Keeping my eyes demurely downcast, I wait a few beats. Then, very softly, I say, "I just have one question."

When they have leaned in very close to hear me, when I have their full and rapt attention, I raise my eyes slowly, batting my lashes. "Who's going to bust my cherry?" I say.

Their laughter washes over me in a wave of sweetness, like the first spark of love.

Back in the office North gives me a list of photographers, telling me to call them for test shots. "Since you want to try modeling," he says, adding gallantly, "tell you what, I'll even set one up for you right now. How's next week?" The toothpick in his mouth bobs up and down like a handshake.

"Great. Thanks," I say. I am beginning to feel a bit frayed around the edges. The flirty, careless girl I'd pretended to be at lunch is wearing rather thin. It is, I realize, a lot of work to act dishy. I need a recess. What I want more than anything is to go home and sleep.

I fiddle with the chipped handle of North's cowboy boot–shaped pencil holder. My stomach is full and the hot day is making me even sleepier. While North makes a phone call, I pop a

piece of gum into my mouth, looking around the walls at the photographs of women. Some of the glass in the frames needed a good
dusting. Who are these women? They are all beautiful, as beautiful
as the women in the headshots in Dr. S—'s office. How had they
ended up here, instead of on a television sitcom or in a movie or on
the pages of a magazine? Had they come from some tiny town in
the middle of nowhere, dreaming of success in Hollywood, before
their hopes had gone in an entirely different direction? Or is this
the future they had always envisioned for themselves? They cup
their breasts in their hands, toss their hair over their shoulders, jut
their lovely asses into the camera. They are all naked. It reminds
me of a place my parents and I used to pass on our way to the airport, a "gentleman's club," it was called. My mother's lip always
curled in disdain at the sign, LIVE NUDES, in glittering, large letters.
"*Live* nudes?" she'd say. "Live nudes as opposed to what? Dead
nudes? Why don't they just say nudes and leave it at that? It's
pretty self-explanatory. You can't be just a *little* bit nude, can you,
just like you can't be just *a little bit* pregnant, or a *tiny bit* dead. I
mean, how stupid! *Live nudes.*" My mother would end by clucking
her tongue at the garish sign and saying something like, "How
sad." Meaning sad for the girls inside, the nudes. I thought it
strange that she could not go by this club without giving a disdainful commentary on the women who worked there.

I bid good-bye to North and the other men, promising to call
after I've gone to my meeting with the photographer next week.
Now that the sugar rush of their attention is beginning to wear off,
I am feeling jittery and sheepish, as if I'd awakened beside someone
with whom I did not recall going to bed.

In my car I yank the wig off my head, toss it onto the passenger
seat. I shake out my short, stiff hair, which has become plastered
down to my skull with sweat. My hair is no more than two inches
long. Why did I cut it? What the hell was I thinking?

Answer: I wasn't.

When I was a little girl, I swore I'd never cut my hair. It wasn't because I thought long hair was feminine, or that I preferred the way I looked with it. No. What I loved was the way it felt when I swung my head from side to side and felt the hair whip around my neck like a wild mane. Like Misty of Chincoteague. Unlike other girls, I didn't want to own a horse or ride a horse. I wanted to be a horse.

What happened to that little girl? What happened to *me?* How did I end up a stranger to myself, an anonymous girl posing for nude pictures, wearing a stolen wig? *What happened?*

I switch on the radio, filling up the hot empty air with noise. I turn the hard lump of chewing gum with my teeth, pushing my tongue into the last bit of prickly flavor in the middle. I wish I hadn't made that comment about my cherry. Are North and the other men laughing at me right now, the silly girl from Hancock Park with the mysterious motives? Why had I acted so foolish? Shine a smidgen of attention my way and I turn into a circus monkey, turning flips and doing tricks and screeching hysterically for more, more, more. I gather the scattered coins of any stranger's admiration and clutch them to me like a beggar.

I am, I realize, afraid of my own desperation. I am afraid of what I will do, who I might become.

On the freeway I press my foot to the accelerator, yearning for the freedom of speed. There is always this moment that occurs when driving on the freeway, I find, when my mind is lulled by the motion of the wheels and I forget that I'm traveling at a very high speed, or any speed at all. I could just be standing still. I am going almost seventy now, but I don't feel it. The world races past my window but it's as if I'm not moving at all. It scares me, the fine line between consciousness and oblivion. One swift jerk of the wheel would direct my car into the cement median. Just one single, careless movement is all it would take. I've always wondered if other drivers feel this, if they are as vigilant as I am, as terrified of losing control.

It occurs to me, then, that it is not the dangers of driving I fear, but myself. It is not my car that I am afraid of losing control of. And what I fear most has, in fact, come true: I cannot predict anymore what I will do, how I will act, or how far I will go in any situation. I am out of control, headed for disaster.

Shaken, the palms of my hands damp and threatening to slip off the steering wheel, I focus all my attention on the road, as if the simple act of keeping my car between the yellow lines can save me.

CHAPTER 23

"I miss you, baby," Hank's voice wheedles into my answering machine. "Where have you been? I keep driving by your apartment, but your car is never there."

My car is not there because I am not there anymore, I think. Hank does not know this; I have kept the same phone number, and I'm sure he is not bold enough to ask my former roommates where I am. I haven't had any contact with him since the night he hit Anita. How long will it be, I wonder, before he stops calling? Will he stop calling? Hank is not the sort of person who picks up signals, who gets discouraged. His messages run the gamut from charming and seductive to gruff and irritable. Sometimes he only booms out, "Where the hell *are* you?" then hangs up.

I have to go back to the old apartment, once, a few weeks after I've left, to pick up a few things I forgot: a scarf I lent Anita, some CDs, a few books. Not wanting to see my old roommates, I call Karen and ask her if I can come over on Tuesday afternoon, when I know that she and Hillary will be at work and Anita will be in class. Karen agrees, reluctantly, to leave a key under the flower pot by the back door for me.

"Just don't forget to put it back," she says curtly.

It is strange to go back there, like looking at remnants of another life. Letting myself in, I hurriedly collect the box in which Karen has put my things and carry it down the back stairs, pushing the door open with my foot.

"Hank!"

He is standing right in front of me, as if he knew all along that I would be there and he has been waiting.

"What are you doing here?" I ask, starting to shake. My mind clicks through the facts: No one is home in the apartment; Hank could easily force me back inside. Should I scream? Sprint for my car?

Hank removes the box from my arms and puts it on the ground. Then he steps closer so that he is just a few inches from my face. "What am I *doing* here?" he says. "What do you think I'm doing here? I came to see you."

"I can't see you right now. It's a bad time. I'm about to go out."

"Just a few minutes," Hank whines, putting his hands on my shoulders and squeezing. "I've missed you, baby. Haven't you missed me?"

"Sure, of course," I say, trying to be casual. "It's been a busy time."

We are inside the door. He keeps pushing, gently but firmly, insistently, so that I am forced to climb the stairs backward.

He's going to rape me, I think. *He's going to make me climb back up the stairs and then we'll be alone in the apartment and he'll rape me.*

My heart is pounding so hard I can hear it in my ears. "I have a doctor's appointment," I stammer. "I'll be late. Anita will be home any minute."

"I just want to say hello," he says. "It's been *weeks.*"

I have no choice but to keep backing up the stairs. Hank keeps his hands on my shoulders, his eyes fixed on mine.

"You're not *avoiding* me, are you?" he says.

"No, no, of course not." We are at the top of the stairs, in the kitchen. Across the hall is my old room; if I can sprint in there, I can lock him out. I turn, ducking out from beneath his grasp in one swift motion, and lunge toward the hall. But my foot catches an extension cord, and I trip and fall.

I am on my butt in my doorway. Hank towers above me. The wind is knocked out of me, or maybe it is panic—I can't get my breath. Without thinking, I pull my knees up to my chest and wrap my arms around my body, covering my head with my hands the way they told you to do during earthquake drills in grammar school.

"Are you all right? Let me help you up." With one large hand, he pulls me to my feet. My legs give out and I start to collapse. But Hank is so strong he doesn't need my cooperation to pull me to my feet. He hoists me up with his hands under my armpits.

This is it, I think, squeezing my eyes shut.

"Hank, please," I say. My voice is tiny.

I feel him grasp the front of my T-shirt and pull. I strain against him with all my strength, my back pressed to the wall.

"Holy shit!" Hank exclaims.

I close my eyes tighter, bracing for a blow.

"Did you get a *boob job?*"

Opening my eyes, I see that he is not, in fact, yanking me by my shirt but rather looking down the front of it at my breasts. His expression is mildly curious, as if he were examining items in a shopping bag.

"I *thought* they looked bigger!" he says, delighted. "When did you get it done?"

"About a month ago." I'm still shaking, but something in Hank's manner tells me he does not intend to hurt me. What, then, does he want?

"They look fan*tas*tic!" Hank is gleeful, practically hopping from foot to foot, like a child eager to open a present. "C'mon, let's see them."

"Not now," I say, pretending modesty. "The scars are still pretty bad."

"Oh, the scars, don't worry about the scars." Releasing me, Hank leans back against the opposite wall, crossing his hands behind his head. Suddenly, we are old friends just shooting the breeze. "The scars fade quickly, trust me. Here, I'll show you something."

"What?" Still wary, I hover in the doorway. Hank pulls aside his shorts. As usual, he doesn't wear underwear.

"I've seen it," I remind him.

He begins to stroke himself into arousal.

"Hank, please," I say. "Not now."

"No, wait," he said. "*This*. See that? That little scar?"

Reluctantly I look, maintaining the small distance between us. There is, I see, a narrow, slightly raised ridge along the base of his penis.

"That's a scar?" I ask.

"Yep! But you'd never know it, right? I had a penile implant!" He says this so proudly that I practically expect him to clap his hands together in delight. "Years ago. You never noticed, did you? You probably just thought I was really well-endowed, right?"

"Uh, yeah, I guess so." Actually, I hadn't thought about it at all.

"No one knows," he says. "In fact, you're one of the only people I've told. It's the best thing I ever did, let me tell you."

I do not know what to say. Am I supposed to be touched by his confession?

"I hope you had a good doctor," he says. "It makes *all* the difference. I had a *great* doctor. The best. Maybe you've heard of him? Bob S—?"

The hairs on my arms rise as though a chill has come into the room.

After a moment, I am able to say, "The name sounds familiar." I wonder if Hank can tell I am shivering.

He adjusts his penis, tucking himself away. "Listen, the real reason I've been so eager to see you is *this*." He reaches into his pocket and unfurls a yellow piece of paper. "Here, take a look. This is something you might be interested in."

I look down at the paper, a flier of some sort which must have been hanging up outdoors, perhaps on a telephone pole. I can see staple marks, and the paper is filthy. It is so grimy that I do not want to touch it.

"Read it," Hank says.

I look down, holding the flier gingerly. In large, bold letters it reads:

MAKE HUGE PROFITS
raising Giant California Superworms!
Worms convert garbage into rich fertilizer.
Easy to raise, fast multipliers!
Grow them in your backyard or garage!

"I know, I know, *worms*, right?" Hank says. "But the truth is, they're really fascinating! And the income potential is fantastic! I just got my starter kit, and they're doing so well, I'm thinking of setting up my own operation."

I look at him. "Worms," I say.

"I know what you're thinking. *Worms,* yuck, right? But they're actually very clean. They're totally self-sufficient. They convert their own waste into food. They're very efficient waste processors."

My head seems now to be bobbing of its own accord. A surreal feeling has come over me.

"I thought of you right away, Hope. You're still looking for a job, right? And we get along so well. We could be partners. A joint partnership-type thing. What do you say?"

"Sure," I say weakly. "Great."

"Come downstairs with me for a second," he says. "I've got one of my worm farms in the car. I'll show you."

Numbly, I follow him down the stairs and out the door.

"They're really something," he calls over his shoulder, scampering ahead of me and opening the door of his battered old Ford Fiesta. He rummages among debris on the backseat, emerging with a large, flat Plexiglas box filled with dirt and crisscrossed with little trails. "Look," he says. "Worms!"

The worms do not appear to be moving. I can see a few of them, thick and sickeningly pinkish-brown, pressed like lips against the Plexiglas wall. "I think they might be dead," I say.

"Shit!" Hank smacks the side of the worm farm, and one of the worms stretches, pressing like a tongue against the glass. "Shit! Oh, *shit!* I shouldn't have left them in the car. Well, it's okay. I'll put them in the front seat so the air conditioner can cool them down."

He reaches in and starts his car, then positions the worm farm upright in the passenger seat, securing it with the seat belt. "Listen. Hope. We can talk about this later, okay? I've got to go, I have an audition. It's big-time! A pilot that's being produced by the *Baywatch* people."

"Great," I say, with all the enthusiasm of a snuffed candle.

"So you'll think about the worms thing? Promise me you'll think about it. It's a win-win proposition."

"I'll think about it," I say. *Please go,* I think.

"Keep that flier. *Think about it.* Let me know, okay? Here's my cell phone number."

He squeezes me to him in a brief, hard hug, startling me, then lets go and gets in the car, furiously rolling down all the windows. The air conditioner roars to life. "Worms can't take the heat!" he shouts.

Without thinking, I climb back up the stairs to the apartment. It is not until I am in the kitchen that I remember, with a shock, that I do not live there anymore.

Standing there, I am overcome with a feeling of emptiness that makes me feel as if my whole insides have been hollowed out, like a carved pumpkin. I look down at the dirty flier, ball it up, and put it in the trash can. My hands feel filthy. I stand at the sink for a long time, scrubbing my hands with the soap and the scouring sponge until they're pink and tender, almost raw.

I go down the hall to Anita's room, open the door, and stand in the fragrant hush. The air smells like her shampoo, clean and girly. I feel a sudden, intense longing, standing there surrounded by Anita's things. I know every inch of this room, each of her small possessions. There, on the dresser, is the picture of Anita accepting the Dairy Princess award. She looks younger, plumper, but otherwise the same. Beside the photo is her rhinestone tiara, which she wears in the picture along with the satin banner. When I'd first met her, Anita had told me proudly about how, checking in at the airport for her flight to L.A., she had her tiara with her. When she set it on the counter, the ticket agent promptly upgraded her to first class. She was so proud of this story. I'd laughed inwardly when she told me, mocking her. It occurs to me, now, that her feelings, and our friendship, were things that I didn't take seriously. It wasn't that I didn't care; it just did not seem possible to me that Anita would really care about me, or our friendship. I didn't give myself that much significance, so I assumed I wouldn't be significant to someone else. But my actions *had* had an effect. I had hurt us both.

Looking down at the wood floor I notice, by Anita's bed, a minute bit of mud that she must have tracked in. I grab a Kleenex off the dresser and pick it up. It strikes me, then, how dusty the whole floor looks. And the dresser. And all Anita's pictures. And her tiara. Even her stereo: All are covered in the powder-fine, beige dust that settles daily over everything in Los Angeles.

I go down the hall to the laundry room and get the mop and bucket, pour in oil soap and hot water, and lug it back down the hall. In Anita's room, I pick the pieces of discarded clothing off the floor and fold them neatly on her bed. Then I start scrubbing.

I have never cleaned so carefully. Getting on my hands and knees, I scour each corner and under the bed, all the places where dirt could linger, unseen. Then I dampen a wad of paper towels and dust every surface in her room, until the glass in the picture frames winks in the light and the top of her dresser reflects back my own shiny face.

Breathing hard, I look around the room. It is spotlessly clean, but something is still not right. It is too late, this effort of mine.

I think of a long-ago afternoon, when I was ten or so, at my grandparents' house. I was wandering around alone upstairs, exploring; my parents and the rest of the family were down in the living room. It was a holiday or family dinner. I felt, as I wandered through the quiet rooms, the same odd, light emptiness I always felt in that huge house, as if I were molecule tiny, insignificant. As if I didn't exist. I was overcome with a fervent desire to *do something*, to leave my mark upon the unwelcoming perfection of the house, to assert my existence.

On the large mahogany desk in my grandfather's study, there was a stack of money, fifties and hundreds. Brand-new, crisp bills. At once enticing and forbidding. After a quick glance around, I jammed a fifty into my pocket.

A sense of elation overtook me, but it was brief, dissolving quickly into guilt. No one ever said anything to me, but every time I was around my grandparents I wondered if they knew.

Standing in Anita's room, I think, *I have hardly changed at all.* The way I felt wandering around my grandparents' house is the same way I felt in the apartment when my roommates were out, living what I imagined to be their full, busy lives. I'm still going through life like a lost child, thinking that everyone else has control over things, waiting for someone to tell me what I should do. I am no longer helpless, but I continue to act helpless. I will do, and have done, just about anything to not feel the old familiar despair. Dr. D—, Dr. R—, Dr. S—, Hank, North: all the men whose eyes I've danced in, trying to find a reflection of myself that flatters. But these empty contacts have only left me feeling emptier. Hiding from real life has not, as I thought it would, kept me from hurting.

I do not want to hurt anymore, but I don't know how *not* to hurt. I do not want to obsess anymore, but I don't know how to break out of the prison of my own head. There is no misery like the misery of being trapped in your own brain. The more I think about my problems, the more tied up in knots I become. I do not want to be alone, or pretend that I am not lonely. I don't want to pretend at all. I want connection and excitement and meaning. I looked for those things in Dr. S—'s office and, for a time, I thought I found them there. A long, long time ago something important inside me got crushed, and that little wounded thing is still in there, tiny, afraid to unfold itself.

I can't do this anymore.

I realize I need help.

CHAPTER 24

It is difficult for me to call my mother and ask if her therapist can give me a referral. Even though I long to reach out to her, and I know that she'll be happy to help, there is a part of me that resists revealing weakness, as if showing even a little bit of vulnerability will cause me to crumble. Besides which, my "self-mutilations" have done just what she predicted: They have made me miserable, left me bereft. I know she will not say *I told you so,* she's not that cruel, and I think she is as eager as I am to reestablish a connection between us. Still, I cannot keep from feeling that I will somehow be devoured by her.

I'm relieved when I get her answering machine, so that I can leave a brief, businesslike message.

My mother calls back shortly, and leaves me a name and number: Ellen Ring, in Westwood. I write it down and stare at it for a long time before calling. She asks me to call her back if I want to "talk," but I do not.

On her answering machine, Ellen sounds young and kind, calm. I like her voice. I explain who I am and ask if she could see me next week. I hope that there will be a message from her this afternoon when I get back from Dr. S—'s office.

A part of me still hopes, each time, that seeing Dr. S—will again somehow magically erase the feeling of hopelessness that shadows my days. But the spell is not so strong as it used to be. I am still attracted to Dr. S—, but there is no denying that the thrill is, though not gone, waning. I can still distract myself with the anticipation of an appointment. I dress thoughtfully, apply my makeup with care, dabbing away the inky smudges of mascara that my shaky hand leaves beneath my eyes. I imagine the moment when Dr. S— will see me, the spark of approval in his eyes.

But it is difficult to look forward to an appointment when I know that I am going to experience real pain. Perhaps this accounts for my lack of enthusiasm. Dr. S— lied to me when he said that after the breast surgery, I would be on auto-pilot. Either he lied, or my body is not cooperating. Capsules of scar tissue are forming daily around each implant, making my breasts painfully hard. Dr. S— has to pop them with his hands; when he squeezes, each little capsule pops with a discernible click, like the bubbles in plastic bubble wrap. He has to squeeze hard, and often he must twist and contort my breasts to get at a difficult capsule. It is, often, excruciating. Bruises bloom on my skin after every visit.

Then, for a week or so after, my breasts are soft again. When I ask Dr. S— why this is happening, he says that each patient is different. This just happens to be my body's rather "aggressive" response to the implants. Apparently my body is vigilant about intrusion in a way I am not. He assures me that this reaction will not last more than a few months, but I have lost whatever faith I had in his promises.

Riding the elevator to his office, I begin to panic. My legs go weak and wobbly beneath me; I am overtaken by a sensation that the elevator ropes will suddenly give way and I will plunge to my death. My face, reflected in the steel door, is pale and shiny with perspiration; my careful makeup application ruined. When the doors open at last and I step out onto the twelfth floor, I am in the throes of an all-out anxiety attack. I must force myself to walk through the double doors into Dr. S—'s waiting room, a place that used to be my safety zone, my haven. Now, even the sight of the familiar pale, embryonic walls is not enough to quell my fear.

Dr. S— is rushed and brisk, distracted. He squeezes my breasts in what seems a painfully perfunctory way, reiterating his hollow promise that I will soon be "on auto-pilot." I thank him, put my shirt on quickly.

Leaving the examining room, I see Dr. S— standing in the hall outside his surgical suite with two young women I've never seen before. I turn away from them and hurry toward the door, longing for the safety of my car, my small apartment.

"Hope!"

I turn, a grin contorting my face.

Dr. S— beckons me over. I make an inane gesture—*me?*—jabbing my finger into my chest. He nods. Yes, you. Reluctantly but automatically, I approach him.

"This is Hope," he says to the women. His tone, I notice, is much more enthusiastic than it had been when the two of us were alone in the exam room. It is his showman's voice, the voice he uses when he has an audience, or when he wants to sell a surgery. "Hope had her breasts done—what?—three months ago?"

"Just about."

He introduces the women to me as his fiancée's cousin and her friend. For an instant my heart darkens reflexively at the word fiancée, but the shadow passes quickly.

"Hope here had a *won*derful result," he says, his voice like poured gravel. Then, turning to me, "You wouldn't mind showing them yours, would you, Hope?"

He can't be serious, I think. He can't be asking me to show them my painful breasts as an example of successful surgery. But then it occurs to me that in spite of everything, my breasts *look* perfectly fine; even, I suppose, beautiful. The bruises will not appear until to-night.

"Do you mind, Hope? It'll just take a second."

"Um, sure. Okay." I hate myself for my passivity, my inability to say no. Why am I so afraid of Dr. S—'s disapproval? I make a mental note to talk about this when I see Ellen Ring. Ellen Ring, with her calm, motherly voice. The thought gives me hope. Maybe after I see Ellen Ring I won't feel as if I have to take my shirt off in front of strangers just because Dr. S— asks me to.

Back in the exam room I sit down on the table while the three of them stand together near the door. The women look uncomfortable; they are smiling, but their arms are crossed protectively over their own chests. It occurs to me that they are perhaps as uncomfortable as I with what is going on. I take off my shirt and bra in front of them, feeling like Exhibit A.

"Just look at those. Those are some boobies, aren't they?" Dr. S—'s gravelly voice is full of pride.

The women nod. *Did he really just say boobies?*

"Doing Hope's breasts changed the way I did breasts forever."

He approaches me, his hands outstretched, a gleam in his eye. "I want to show these ladies something," he says.

I am unprepared for what happens next.

Dr. S— begins to play with my breasts as if they are not attached to my body. He squeezes and manipulates them, holding one in each hand, alternately pushing up one and then the other and letting each drop with a jiggle, the way a child might practice at juggling. He does this for, it seems, minutes, accompanying his fondling with a murky, verbose commentary about age and skin elasticity which makes no sense at all.

I try to meet the eyes of the women, to gauge their reaction; each is looking intently at Dr. S— and nodding as solemnly as if she were in a college lecture hall. I look down to my sore, inflated breasts in his hands and feel a dull horror.

"I've got to go," I say, shrugging out from under his touch.

Dr. S— looks down at his empty hands with surprise, like a

child who's just had his cookie taken away. He recovers quickly, smoothly.

"In fact," he says to his fiancée's cousin, "*this* is how I'm going to do Margo's breasts."

Margo, his fiancée. Of course. He is going to augment Margo's breasts. Even the woman he loves is not perfect enough for him.

I reach for my shirt. As I shift on the table, my thighs unstick from the vinyl with a long smack.

Dr. S— and the two women leave, and I dress again, quickly, and slip out of the room. They are standing in the hall outside the surgical suite when I come out.

The door to one of the other exam rooms opens then, and a young woman in a green surgical gown steps out. She looks pale and frightened, but she smiles when she sees Dr. S—.

"Tina!" Dr. S— beams at her.

She can't be more than twenty-two. There are dark shadows beneath her pale blue eyes, as if she spent a sleepless night.

"Ready?" he asks.

Tina blushes and nods, as Dr. S— turns his full mega-watt charm on for her. It is like watching someone fire up a furnace.

"Listen. I have a surprise. These ladies are going to watch your surgery today!" With a casual sweep of his hand, he gestures toward the fiancée's cousin and her friend. The way he says it—*watch your surgery today*—makes it sound like something special, a privilege.

Tina's face betrays surprise, but she smiles. "Okay," she says uncertainly.

"I was just saying, Tina, how Hope here"—he shoots his thumb at me—"had a fan*tas*tic result. One of my best ever."

Tina murmurs something like, "Oh! Good." Her feet in their paper booties shuffle soundlessly on the linoleum floor.

Dr. S— turns to me, waiting for my endorsement.

"Well? Hope? You *are* happy with your result, right? *Tell* her." There is an undertone of angry impatience in Dr. S—'s tone. He tries to hide it with his wide, dazzling smile.

Words are bubbling up inside my head, words that will not

come out. I want to smack the side of my head with my hand so that they will spill out of my mouth. *Don't do this,* I want to say to her. *Don't do it, don't do it, don't do it.*

"You *did* get what you wanted, didn't you?" Dr. S—'s brown eyes have turned hard and impenetrable.

Say something! I shout at myself. *Tell Dr. S— that it isn't all right for him to use your surgery to impress these women. Speak up!*

For the first time I can recall, the office is silent. Tina and I look at each other. She blinks, hopeful, uncertain. She is waiting for me to say something that will reassure her that she is doing the right thing. She is so young.

I am, I feel, looking at myself.

Dr. S—'s glare is unbearable. Quietly, I say, "I got what I asked for."

Dr. S— raises his eyebrows at me in surprise; obviously, I have not given the response he wanted. He turns toward the three women so that they can see his incredulous look. "I should *hope* so," he says curtly. "Considering, let's see, *how* many times have you been here in the past months?"

"Um, I . . . I don't know." Caught off-guard, I stammer. "I didn't exactly—"

"She practically *lives* here." Dr. S— laughs through his nose, like a horse.

Startled, I take a step back. The room quivers; the white walls, floor, ceiling blend together. "I've been here a lot, yes, that's true, but all your patient—"

"This girl is my *number one* fan!" he bellows. "I can't get her out of my office!"

Tears have formed in my eyes, blurring my vision. I blink them back.

The three women have started to giggle tentatively, nervously. Dr. S—, sensing an appreciative audience, warms to his material. He turns to Tina.

"If you knew how often she was here, you'd think I should be charging her rent!"

My mouth falls open. Tina gives a short, sharp laugh, relieved, probably, to be distracted from her own fear.

"What can I do?" Dr. S— cries, tossing his hands in the air in mock exasperation. "She just won't *leave!*"

"That's not fair," I murmur, trying to keep my chin from trembling. "How can you—"

"Ah, listen." Dr. S— grabs me to him, wrapping an arm around my shoulders and rattling me against him so hard my teeth click together. "I'm teasing, you know that, right? Of *course* I like having you around here. She's beautiful, isn't she?"

The three women nod obediently, in unison.

"I made her that way." Dr. S— releases his hold on me and turns toward his rapt audience. "I have that effect on women. Every woman I've ever known has improved herself in some way, and not just physically. Margo got that big promotion just weeks after we met, and now she's . . ."

I turn, already knowing the rest of his story. As I push through the door, I glance back at Tina, feeling a stab of guilt. But would anything I say really change her mind? Would a stranger's words of warning have changed *mine?*

No.

As I close the door behind me, Dr. S—, the ringmaster, is ushering the three women toward his surgical suite with a gallant sweep of his arm.

"And now, if you'll follow me, ladies," he's saying.

Waiting for the elevator, I wrap my arms around my body. I'm shivering, though not from cold. I feel like I am drifting up and out of my body.

In the supermarket the other day, I ran into a girl from my high school class, Bradford Banning. In my usual state of panic, I was hurrying, stuffing fruits and vegetables into my basket. I pretended not to see her. But she was staring at me.

"Hope?"

"Yes? Oh, Bradford! Hi. I didn't recognize you."

She was staring so intently at me I felt as if I might drop the melon I was holding, shattering its fragile contents on the floor. "*I didn't* recognize *you*," she said. "You look a bit . . . have you lost weight?"

"Um, no." *My face is more angular because I've had surgery.* Then I remembered something people who are post–plastic surgery often say to deflect attention from the changes they've made in themselves. "I cut my hair," I said.

"Yes. I see. But it's just that . . . you . . ." She shook her head, remembering her manners. "Sorry. I didn't mean to be rude. People change so much after high school, don't they? I wasn't sure that was you. I was trying to remember whether you had an older sister."

"I don't," I said.

"Right. Well, it's good to see you." She touched nervously at her black velvet hair band. "So what are you up to these days?"

I mumbled the usual inanities about looking for a job. "In fact, I'm late for an interview now," I said. My panic was starting, making the floor beneath me feel uncertain. "I'm sorry, I'd love to chat, but—"

"No, no, you go. See you later."

I was so relieved to be out from under her inspection that I went straight home. I didn't even think about the incident.

Now, waiting for the elevator, I think, *Have I really changed myself that much?* It didn't seem so to me, but then I'd watched my face change in increments. Is it possible that someone like Bradford really wouldn't recognize me because of all the surgeries? I wanted to transform myself, to shed my skin and become someone else entirely. But now, the realization of what I've done fills me with dread. Have I lost all traces of myself? Did I really want to lose that girl completely? Was she so hideous? Is it too late?

The elevator doors part, a great mouth opening wide for me. I step in as if in a dream, vaguely aware that the other people inside step silently back and away from me as I enter, clearing a space for the young woman getting on who must look as if she's just seen a ghost.

CHAPTER 25

I'm driving down a wide, empty street in Van Nuys bordered by decrepit houses when I pull over to study North's directions. A long, low black Cadillac cruises by me, its windows tinted black, emitting thumping music so loud it vibrates my car. Gangbangers, I think. My heart skips with panic. I hold my breath as the car drives slowly past.

I am shaking when I finally find the address North gave me, one of several low stucco buildings that look as unassuming as garages or storage sheds, plain with just the street numbers painted on them huge and black. I park my car in a narrow wedge of shade and get out, smoothing down my sundress. Taking a breath, I knock firmly on the door.

A slight, gray-haired man answers. He blinks in the bright light; he looks as if he might have been napping. Behind him the space yawns dark and vast as a cave.

"North's girl?" he asks.

"Yes."

I follow him into the studio, with its bare gray walls, where I can barely make out a camera on a tripod with a cloth thrown over it. He shuts the door behind us, eliminating the slash of bright out-door light, and for a moment, while my eyes adjust, I am unable to see, and feel a flash of panic.

The photographer, who says his name is George, is loading film into a Polaroid camera. He is wearing a blue button-down shirt and jeans. His thin gray hair is combed back. He looks like someone's grandfather.

"Go ahead and take off your clothes," he says. "You can stand right there."

My fingers reach up to undo the buttons of my dress. I feel as if I am not really in my body. I have felt this way since this morning, when I could not decide whether or not to go to this appointment. Something told me not to go, but something pushed me out the door, a vague memory of the thrill I felt in North's office. And there is the possibility, too, that after this initial meeting, I may be hired to pose for this photographer. One thousand to twenty-five hundred dollars a day: That was the amount of money I could earn in a day, North said, for nude pictures.

The dress slips to the floor around my feet. My fingers reach around to undo my bra; my panties slip down my legs. I feel, stand-ing naked before the photographer, as if I am lightly dozing. It is comforting, this familiar numbness. Like a cocoon.

The camera flashes. In between each bright explosion, the rest of the room swims into focus. "What's that?" I ask, noticing several ropes and straps hanging from the ceiling. "And *that?*" Something that looked like a horse's harness is slung over a chair.

"That's for the bondage work. Do you mind uncrossing your arms? I can't see your body."

I realize I am holding my arms around my body, as if I were cold.

The photographer pauses, looking at me. "North didn't tell you? That's what I do. Bondage shots."

When I don't speak, he adds, "I can show you some of my pictures, if you want. Give you a better idea."

Maybe I nod, or my head bobs involuntarily, because he pulls a few black-and-white photographs from inside a battered metal desk and hands them to me. "This is what we're aiming for," he says.

The image in the photograph won't quite come into focus. I turn it this way and that. Finally, I manage to stammer, "I think I've got this one upside down. Is she supposed to be hanging like this?"

"Yep. You've got it right. It's not really painful. We take you down between shots."

I flip to the next photograph. "Oh, my God."

The woman in the photograph is on her knees, her hands tied behind her back. She is blindfolded. She wears only a black G-string. Her mouth is open, stretched wide, and there is a knife on her tongue. The handle sticks out of her mouth, the paper-thin blade rests atop her tongue like a communion wafer.

My God, I think. *My God, this is not right. Ca n'existe pas.* For some reason, my mind switches gears and I am suddenly, inexplicably thinking in French, just as I did years ago, putting what is unthinkable and inexpressible into a foreign language. *Elle a un couteau sur la langue. Elle va se couper.* She has a knife on her tongue. She is going to cut herself.

My hands shake visibly as I hand the pictures back to the photographer.

"Are you all right?" he asks.

I nod, feeling dizzy.

"Okay," he says.

The flash explodes again, like an assault, disorienting me.

Suddenly, I am not in the photographer's studio anymore. I am sixteen years old, listening to my mother's screams. The horror of it dawns on me as I look down at my naked body; I am *her,* I am the girl my father can't sit next to, the scantily clad seductress. *Flash.* The gray walls of the studio become the muted colors of

Camille's office. I am there with my mother, confused but determined, prepared to say that my father molested me. I will say anything, anything at all to win her. My mouth is full of lies. I will invent any dark secret; I will shift shape into any form; I will betray not only my father but myself, if only she will love me. But my mother's stare is ice. As she slams the door, I know I have been tricked. I have offered her everything, just so that she can tell me, again, I am nothing. I am humiliated, exposed, stripped naked. *Flash.* My chest fills up with a sob; I want to hide from the shame of it, the shame of *me.* No time has passed at all. I am that girl, and I am here now, she and I are one. Both of us implore, *See me. Love me. Want me.*

　　Flash.

　　And then, somehow, it is as if I wake up.

　　I reach for my dress, yank it off the floor to cover myself. "I'm sorry," I say. "I can't do this. I'm sorry I wasted your time." *There is no amount of money in the world that would make me do this,* I think. It is the first definite thought I've had in months, perhaps years, and the clarity with which it presents itself in my head makes me feel giddy.

　　George puts down his camera. I expect him to be annoyed with me. But he does not look angry, or even surprised. He just looks old.

　　"Not everyone is cut out to do this," he says.

　　I fumble the dress over my head, pull on the panties, hold the bra balled up in my hand. All I want to do is get out of here. Dust from the floor clings to the fabric; I can feel it against my skin, each little grain like sandpaper. Yet I am filled with such sudden, overwhelming relief that I want to laugh out loud. "I made a mistake," I say. "I made a mistake."

　　"You're young enough to make mistakes," George says.

　　He pulls the last Polaroid through the camera. I wonder: Does he have a daughter of his own, or a granddaughter, and does he ever see them in the young, desperate women like me whom he photographs?

"Sometimes I get other work," he says, tapping the Polaroids into a neat pile in his hand. His voice is wistful, resigned. "But people like this type of thing. Men like it. There's a big demand for it. Do you want your Polaroids?"

I am about to say no, but the thought of naked pictures of myself lying in a trash can disturbs me. "Please," I say.

"Here."

I look at myself in the pictures and am surprised by how young I look, and how eager. Except for the fact that I'm naked, I could be posing for my college yearbook picture. I'm wearing the wig, which looks almost like my own hair did in college; it spills over my bare breasts, one nipple blooming through the long strands like a pale pink rosebud. I am smiling broadly and unself-consciously, and I am, I think with wonder, beautiful.

"Not bad, huh?" says George, the photographer. "Give them to your boyfriend."

I stare in awe at the Polaroid. What I see astonishes me: a young, lovely, seemingly uncomplicated woman, not at all the despairing, unattractive person I see every day. It occurs to me, then, just how much my inner feelings color the way I see the outside of myself.

I stare and stare at the Polaroid, until the woman in it seems unknowable, someone to whom I bear only a physical resemblance, nothing more. *I have become a stranger to myself,* I think. A beautiful stranger.

"Here." The photographer picks up my purse from the floor, pats off the dust and hands it to me, a small, unexpected gesture of kindness that makes me want to cry.

"Thank you," I say. I stuff the Polaroids in my purse and walk out the door.

Inside my apartment the answering machine shows two messages. The first is Ellen Ring, the therapist, confirming our appointment

for the following week. The second is from a temp agency that I'd
signed up with a week ago. I did not know, as I took the typing test
and talked with the woman behind the desk, whether I'd have the
courage to actually go to any job they might find for me, but I had
forced myself to act as if I would. Now they have a job for me, the
very next day, as a receptionist at a Japanese animation company in
Glendale. It is a temporary position but with long-term potential
and room for advancement. A young, creative environment. I am
to see a Miss McManus at eight in the morning. Can I please call
back and confirm that I will, in fact, be available tomorrow?

A shock of fear shoots through me. Why am I so terrified of this
most ordinary challenge—answering phones, typing some papers—
which I can surely master? I know what it is: I am afraid that I will
disappoint everyone. I am afraid that I can't do it, that I don't have
the energy. Why is it that I'm willing to go to an unknown photographer's studio, and yet I am terrified of a simple temp job? Normalcy scares me. I feel, somehow, that I have failed at life, or that I
am bound to fail. I am afraid that I will collapse under the weight of
any responsibility placed on me.

You can do this, I tell myself. *Just try it. How much harder can it
be than all the other crazy things you've put yourself through?*

I play through the message again, writing it down. I cannot
shake this feeling of dread. But then I think of something Ellen
Ring told me at our first session last week: It is possible to feel terrified and panicky about something and to do it anyway. Feelings
are not reality. Just because I *feel* like I might faint or crumble in a
situation doesn't mean that I will. It was astonishing how comfortable I felt in Ellen's office. I poured out my story to her, barely
pausing for breath. There was no judgment in her eyes. Even when
I pushed her to judge me, even when I asked, "So do you think I'm
a terrible person?" She shook her head. "Why would I think you're
a terrible person?" she said. "You're a confused person, that's all.
But there's nothing terrible about that." Ellen pointed out that I
tend to approach everything from an emotional standpoint; I must

learn to use my mind more, to *think* instead of blindly reacting. Now, I look at the paper with the job information on it and think, *The dread and anticipation I feel thinking about the job are probably much worse than the job itself will be.*

My cat, Henry, snakes his tail around my legs, and I shake some kibble in his dish. It occurs to me that I feel as lost and aimless in my apartment as I do out in the world. Being alone is no longer a safety zone for me. I walk to the bookshelf and switch on the old metal fan I'd bought at a garage sale that roars like a chainsaw. I sit down on the bed beside the little electric fireplace with the fake coals which glows a surreal red and orange when you flip a switch but does not emit any heat. How silly, to have a fireplace, fake or otherwise, in a tiny studio apartment in Los Angeles. The apartment is so small that, sitting on the end of my bed, I can rest my feet flat against the opposite wall. It seems, I think, a metaphor for how small and shrunken and confining my life has become. I have, quite literally, boxed myself in. If I want to spread out, if I want to stretch, I'll have to go outside of these four familiar walls.

Miss McManus. Eight a.m. I fold the paper in half and put it in my purse, where the Polaroids edge their way out of a side pocket. *What are you saving* these *for?* I think, disgusted. I throw them into the trash can.

Outside my window, the late-afternoon sun has a strange intensity. Perhaps it is the broth of smog that makes the light coming through my window the color of a flame. I go to the window and stare at the sun as it pours, liquid, over the old Spanish houses across the street. All day a haze has hung over the city; now, in the last moments before dusk, the sun has finally and brilliantly asserted itself. It occurs to me that what I have been living up until now is an imitation of life. I am, at last, ready to break out from my limited, artificial world into something bigger, brighter, something real.

I go back over to the trash. The Polaroids are resting atop an empty can of tuna. I take one out and wipe off the smudge of grease with a paper towel. I look at the girl smiling back at me. I want to condemn her and her actions, to throw her out, bury her under the rubbish and debris like something shameful. But I have spent my life so cavalierly rejecting parts of myself, deftly slicing out the areas that seemed unworthy, unacceptable, until there is nearly nothing left. I have cut myself up more than any surgeon: *This part is good, this one here is bad; this one needs improvement.* The girl in the Polaroid is me, a part of me that I'll leave in the past, yes, but a part of me nonetheless. If I can learn to feel compassion for myself and my mistakes, perhaps I can learn to forgive both myself and others.

As evening draws the last light from the sky, and the sun at last surrenders itself, I put the photograph in a drawer by my bed. It is one of the places where I keep small things I don't feel like looking at anymore, but am not yet willing to throw away.

CHAPTER 26

Periods of peace are no less interesting than periods of chaos, but they may seem so in the retelling. What can I say about this period, when my life became calm in ways I'd not known before?

The only way I knew to change how I felt about myself was to change my appearance. But now, I am learning to change from the inside out. In Ellen's office, I discover a me that is far different than what I think of myself. The young woman sitting on Ellen's couch is likeable, funny, smart. I marvel at this woman until gradually, I begin to feel like her. I begin to see that she is me.

My father accepted a vice chairman position at a major East Coast bank, and my parents have moved to Pennsylvania. My mother and I talk on the phone, at first every couple of weeks, then, as we become less tentative, more frequently. It seems that the distance between us is helpful as we mend things between us. Not having to look directly at one another allows us to speak more freely and unself-consciously; we do not talk about the past, but we talk, once again, with the ease of girlfriends, eager to hear each other's news. We say *I love you, I miss you*, the phone giving us the privacy we need to express these feelings.

Every day I go to work at the Japanese animation company. It's a short commute over the Hollywood Hills to Glendale, a sleepy suburb of Los Angeles. I like—I find that I need, in fact—the routine of getting up early each morning and having somewhere to go. It's a small company, with just ten employees, and I enjoy the familial atmosphere. I do my job very well and am perceived as competent and capable. After working there for three months, the company president offers me a permanent position as office manager. I accept it, knowing that this is not what I want to do for the rest of my life, but for now, I'm grateful. I've worked out payment plans with the credit card collection agencies, though my credit is so damaged I will have to wait the requisite seven years before I can apply for another card.

I've begun to write again, long letters to old friends, as well as bits of short stories. I write about my former roommates, about Hank, about Dr. S—, filling yellow legal pad after legal pad on my lunch break and in the evenings. It's as if I'm trying to expunge something, or make sense of it all.

I'm not obsessing nearly as much on my looks; I change my hair color a few times, but that is the extent of it. In therapy I make very quick progress, which Ellen attributes to my readiness to change. "When someone wants to get better, they get better," she says, which makes me think of a quote I once heard: "When the student is ready, the teacher appears." Ellen and I talk about the surgeries I've had. The one I most regret is my breasts. My natural breasts were perfectly fine; they were beautiful. When Dr. S— asked me, "Bigger or smaller?" that should have told me right there that I didn't need implants. But I couldn't see what other people saw. I was not able to see what I had, only what I wanted, what I thought I lacked. Now, my breasts are too big and heavy, making me self-conscious and uncomfortable. I am constantly aware of having two large, fake appendages on the front of my body. I tell Ellen how often I reproach myself for having the implants put in. *How stupid I was,* I say, but Ellen stops me, reminding me to be gentler on myself, less judgmental. Together we work on my tendency toward perfectionism, my habit of heaping criticism upon myself. I am, without doubt, my harshest critic. It is something Ellen says she sees often in her female clients, particularly in regard to their looks.

At work, I've formed a friendship with one of the executives, Ray Donahue. We have a lot in common, though our backgrounds could not be more different. He grew up in New Jersey, the son of a police detective. His big, Irish-Italian family is close, loud, and outspoken. Like me, he lived overseas, spending four years in Sydney, Australia. Ray is entirely self-made, the first in his family to go to college, to hold a white-collar job. We are both homebodies, we have a similar sense of humor, we've read the same books and loved the same movies. There is, from the start, an attraction between us, but one we do not initially act upon, both of us wary of dating a co-worker in such a small office.

When we begin dating, things between us progress quickly. Almost immediately, we are spending all our free time together. We talk about my moving into his house in the Hollywood Hills, since I am there so much anyway. I had always feared a "normal" relationship the same way I'd feared a job. Normalcy, to me, meant complacency and boredom. But my relationship with Ray is remarkably without drama, yet no less intoxicating. We cook dinners together, take hikes, make love. My heart flips over when I see him the way it did for other boyfriends, without the crushing sadness or cruelty or neediness which marred those relationships. I've always thought I had to pay for happiness with an equal measure of suffering. But I'm realizing that this is not the case. Perhaps I just feel more deserving.

Ray is eleven years older than me, never married, having devoted himself entirely to his career. He is very open about the fact that he wants a family. When he mentions us getting married, I freeze up inside. I love him, but things are not moving as quickly for me. His certainty brings up my doubts, and I fear I may never be able to make the decision to get married and have children because I am so fickle. My feelings change from one moment to the next. I have a tendency to get myself into situations and relationships and then feel trapped by them. I'm afraid of my own inconstancy.

Even after the months of therapy, I still have enough self-doubt that other people's desires and decisions seem more valid to me than my own. Ray drops hints about my getting pregnant. When he finds my birth control pills, he scolds me about how bad they are for me. I know the message he's sending: Just stop taking them. And I'm tempted. It seems such an easy solution: Just get pregnant. So much uncertainty in my life will be solved by this. Won't it? I begin to obsess over this the way I obsessed over each surgery. It seems that the only way to get out of my confusion is to just go ahead and get pregnant. I can't quite make the decision to stop taking the pills altogether, but I become careless about missing a pill here and there. *Let Mother Nature decide,* I think. *I can't.*

Sure enough, five months after my twenty-fifth birthday, I find out that I'm pregnant.

Ray is thrilled; he wants to get married at once, but I cannot match either his joy or his conviction. In spite of the fact that it is not a total surprise, I feel overwhelmed, paralyzed with doubt. I have never been confident at my ability to make a decision, and this monumental one feels overwhelming, even though I am the one who put myself in the position of having to make it. Thrown into emotional turmoil, I sink back into a depression. I cannot tell what it is I want. I cry often, and Ray is there for me, reassuring me that we will do whatever it is I want. We don't have to have the baby, he says. But ironically, having the baby is the one thing I'm sure of. I do not doubt even for an instant that I want this child, and my certainty about this awes me. It is my role in all of this that I doubt: What if I fail as a wife, as a mother? The consequences of this decision are so much greater than those of any I've made before. With a surgery, the only risk I was taking was to myself. Now, there are two other lives at stake, Ray's and our child's. If I fail at this, my failure will be disastrous not only to myself but to them.

All of my old fears and phobias rush back in. I've always been terrified of leaving a mark, any mark upon the world. Ellen calms me, helps me talk through my tangled feelings. My anxiety, which has been at bay these past months, comes back with a vengeance. Some days, I can barely make it to her office. My despair is so profound that I am unable to go to work. Impulsively, I quit, give notice on my apartment, and tell Ray that I am moving into his house and that he must take care of me. He is, naturally, both angered at my refusal to consult him about my decision and baffled by the inertia I've settled into. This is a side of me he's never seen. But even though I've lost confidence in myself, he never loses confidence in me.

I'm aware of falling back into my old patterns of helplessness and confusion, but I'm unable to stop myself. I just want to sleep until I feel able to wake up and claim my life. In Ellen's office, I tell her that this pregnancy feels like something that *happened* to me, not something I chose for myself, though I know that this is not true. I feel like I've enrolled in a crash course called Taking Responsibility for My Life and My Decisions. Creating a child seems like something too huge and scary for me to claim responsibility for. Ellen and I talk a lot about my not feeling "big" enough to fill my life. It's how I felt at Berkeley: so light and insignificant, gravity itself could not hold me to the ground. Gradually, the more I talk to Ellen, a thaw begins inside me. It's like being able to feel again after being numb.

When I am six weeks pregnant, Ray and I go together to my first ultrasound. There, on the screen, amid the small, mysterious grayish mass, is the tiny, quicksilver heart. I squeeze Ray's hand, full of hope and fear.

We decide to elope to Las Vegas to get married. I have never been one to fantasize about a big, elaborate wedding, and I feel even less enthusiastic about it now. Having only just accepted that this is what I want, I don't feel ready to share my tentative joy with a lot of other people. I have, as yet, only a fragile faith in my decision, and I fear the scrutiny of a big event at which I will be the focus. The times in my life when I've been in the spotlight are times I've felt false, disconnected from myself, as if I had to perform. I don't want my wedding to be like that.

My parents fly from Pittsburgh to Las Vegas for the ceremony. They are disappointed that I won't be having a big wedding, but they are supportive. In Las Vegas, the surreal atmosphere contributes to the feeling of unreality I have. On the surface, I am calm and relaxed. I blame my overwhelming fatigue on my pregnancy. I even joke with Ray: Should we get married by a pirate, an Elvis impersonator, or Merlin the magician? Inside, I am somnambulant. We stroll through the endless artificially lit arcades and casinos, unable to tell if it is day or night. I am glad for the buzz of noise and activity around us, for it seems to compensate for the energy I lack. We wander around, staring at spectacle after spectacle. There is no need for action on my part, only reaction. I wonder if this is part of the reason people come here, to be freed from the pressure of initiative and action. It is a place of permanent distraction. You are entertained whether you want to be or not. The only static in your brain is the constant ringing and whirring of slot machines.

Inside a dome in the arcade at Caesar's Palace, we gape open-mouthed at the laughing, cavorting Greek gods, brought to life by the magic of lasers. Dionysius raises a glass to his lips and his abundant belly jiggles with mirth. My mother and I buy matching earrings, dangling shards of phosphorescent glass which we are told is the same material space shuttles are made of. Inside Treasure Island, I am drawn back again and again to the white tigers pacing in their glass enclosure. Lounging on their plastic rocks, they unfurl massive paws and stare with languid boredom at the tourists gaping at them. *How is it,* I wonder, *that they are able to feel so at ease, in this atmosphere of manufactured comfort?*

After the marriage ceremony, performed not by someone in costume but by a priest, we have prawn cocktails and champagne in my parents' suite. I hold a small curved prawn to my abdomen and say, *It's about that size now, isn't it?* It is the first time I've spoken directly about the baby.

Slowly, over the following months, I feel better. It is a wonderful surprise to find that I love being pregnant, love the changes in my body and the freedom which pregnancy brings. It's as if, full of a greater purpose, I have permission to stop obsessing about my looks. I feel free to marvel at my newly plump face and changing body without having to think about what is wrong with it. The neurotic patter in my head stops almost entirely. Everything I do and think is geared toward the baby, and it is a huge relief, a gift, this necessary selflessness. Caught up in the excitement of prenatal visits, baby showers, and newly married life, I am delighted, busy, whole.

Nicholas arrives late one hot August night, his birth easy and miraculous. When the nurse hands him to me, the first thing I do is to press my nose to his tiny head, inhaling his baby scent. It is a mother-animal reaction, wholly instinctive. I know, instantly, that I will recognize his smell, his cry, from any other baby's. While Ray goes with the nurse to assist in Nicholas's first bath, I sit up in my hospital bed and call my parents, who will be arriving from Pittsburgh in two days. It is the middle of the night, but they answer on the first ring. "He's here," I say. "He's so beautiful." Contentment flows through my body the way milk flows from my breasts, abundantly. I am full, bountiful, a woman.

I do not go back to work. I do not want to. With Ray's support, I stay home to take care of Nicholas. I pack him up and take him to Ellen's office with me. At home, I put him in his stroller and we take long walks around the Hollywood Hills. Nicholas has mild jaundice, for which the doctor prescribes sunlight that has been filtered through a window, so we spend hours lying on the carpet by the plate-glass window in the living room, soaking up the sun. Motherhood comes naturally to me, filling me with joy and confidence.

Caught up in a passionate love affair with my son, I do not realize
how isolated I've become. I do not see anything obsessive in how
all-consuming my solitude is. I go for days without conversing with
another adult except for Ray or Ellen. I walk back and forth to
Nicholas's crib, watching his sleeping face, waiting for him to wake
up. It just doesn't seem worth the trouble of trying to get out the
door with all the baby gear. I don't acknowledge the possibility that
I'm using motherhood as an excuse to cut myself off from the
world. With both Ray and Ellen, I pretend that I am busier than I
really am. And I *am* content, more so than I've ever been. I'm
happy lying on the couch all day with my son on my chest, nursing
and dozing. Why, I think, do I want to go out, when everything I
need is right here?

Meanwhile, Ray has taken a job with a major television studio
in Westwood. His commute and his hours are much longer than
before. Some days, I'm alone for fifteen hours at a stretch. I'm embarrassed to tell Ray just how isolated I've allowed myself to become. I call it post-partum blues and hope it will pass. Inside me,
something is faltering. I've begun running to the mirror again, perhaps forty, fifty times a day, checking, scrutinizing. My nose, I
think, could be a bit slimmer; my lips could be fuller. When I share
some of my obsessing with Ray, he doesn't understand. He tells me
to find a hobby. His sister, he says, makes jam. Why don't I do
something like that? Stung by his easy dismissal of my problem, I
shut down. I feel even more ashamed: it's my own fault that I'm
obsessing again, that I'm lonely; why don't I make more of an effort to keep busy, to get out and meet other mothers? What is
wrong with me?

I talk about it with Ellen, but in spite of the progress I've made
in her office, the longing inside me, the little voice demanding that
I change myself, does not go away this time. Vague, gnawing, it is
always there, like hunger pains. There is one thing I want to do,
and that is to see Dr. S——. I want to talk to him about my nose, and
I also want that feeling of purpose and excitement I used to get in

his office, the thrill of his attention. One morning, when the weight of silence in the house threatens to overwhelm me, I call his office and book an appointment for the next day. I am so embarrassed, I do not tell either Ellen or Ray about it.

Insight, I realize, is not always a balm for my suffering.

CHAPTER 27

After two years, Dr. S——'s waiting room has not changed. I have to struggle a little getting through the door, because I am pushing a stroller with my six-month-old son, Nicholas, in it. There, right away, is the same papier-mâché puffer fish on a stand in one corner. The aquatic green walls. The sturdy teak coffee table is still stacked with magazines and large, glossy books of photography. I write my name on the sign-in sheet—this is new—and then maneuver the stroller to an available space at one end of the green sectional sofa, upon which three other patients, a man and two women, already sit this morning. None of them look up from their magazines at us, save for the woman who has to move over slightly to make room for me to sit. As she glances up, I smile at her, and she smiles back. Her smile is furtive, a bit startled, and it disappears again quickly behind the mask of impassivity which the other patients wear. It is a look I know well, one which I used to wear myself. I realize I have forgotten the unspoken code: No one looks at each other in a plastic surgeon's waiting room.

Nicholas gurgles and coos, and I pull his plastic teething rattle out of the diaper bag and hand it to him, overly conscious of the sound it makes in the quiet room. Leaning over him, I murmur into his neck, nuzzle my face into the shampoo smell of his wispy baby hair, aware that I'm trying too hard, putting on a show of motherly love for the strangers in the waiting room, as if by demonstrating to them what a good mother I am, I will somehow convince myself. I feel terrible about being back here, even worse for bringing my son with me. I can't help feeling as if I'll damage him by bringing him to this place I used to come to when I was so damaged. Since leaving home this morning, my feelings have been so conflicted that I feel as if I'm sitting here with only half my brain. In my car I'd felt so distracted, I worried that I shouldn't be driving. It's the worst feeling, this confusion. It's agony. I'm acting against my better judgment, unable or simply unwilling to stop myself from doing so. I can't believe I used to feel this way every day, all the time.

I debate getting up and walking back out the door. But before I can, another door opens, the one separating the waiting room from the rest of the office. To my surprise, it is not the receptionist but Dr. S— himself who stands there. He is smiling, still handsome, though there is something slightly different about him. As if no time at all has passed, I feel the old familiar jolt of attraction, the way your stomach seems to drop out of you on a roller coaster.

He wears an eager expression today, like a rock star sneaking a peek at the crowd of fans assembled to see him. When his eyes fall on me, he does a sort of double-take. "It's you!" he says. Then: "Is it you?"

"It's me," I say, warmed by his attention. Then it occurs to me that he may have forgotten my name. "It's Hope."

"You look fantastic," Dr. S— says. "Hope." Something about the way he says my name makes me think he is doing one of those word-association games in his head. He looks from me to the stroller. "Is that your baby?"

"Yes," I say proudly, fussing with the appliquéd frog bib around his neck. "He's almost seven months old. He's—" I look up. Where is Dr. S—? Dr. S— has disappeared. I am talking to an empty doorway.

I sit on the couch, frustrated not with Dr. S— but with myself. Why would I expect Dr. S— to genuinely be interested in my child?

Another patient is called into the office. *I can get up and walk out of here,* I think for the hundredth time, looking at Nicholas. *I can leave.* It can't be worth it, can it, all this effort and agonizing, deceiving my husband (I feel like I've deceived him, by not telling him where I am), all for something so silly? I don't, deep down, really want to have my nose done. I have, at best, only a mild interest in the procedure I intend to ask Dr. S— about. What I want is to put an end to the voices in my head, the ones that make me go back and forth to the mirror. Awash in my anxiety, I want someone to throw me a line. Dr. S—'s attention as electric shock therapy—something to jolt me out of the lethargy I'm mired in. But will it be enough to have Dr. S— shine his attention on me and tell me I'm pretty?

"Miss Williams? Mr. Wells?"

The receptionist stands in the doorway, calling two more patients into the office. They practically bolt off the couch, their indifferent expressions melting away at the imminent possibility of a private audience with Dr. S—. To me, the receptionist says, "He'll be right with you." With a start, I recognize her. She is the cousin of Dr. S—'s fiancée, one of the women whom Dr. S— asked me to show my breasts to. She and her friend were going to watch him perform a breast augmentation.

Nicholas has stopped fussing and has fallen asleep in his stroller, his head lolled back, his soft shiny mouth slipping open. I feel a rush of tenderness toward him, and tears rise in my eyes. *Shame on you,* a little voice in my head says. *Bringing an innocent little baby to a plastic surgeon's office!*

"Mrs. Donahue?"

Perhaps the reason the receptionist does not recognize me is because I have a different last name, though I don't think that's it. Considering the intimacy of our last contact, I half expect that she would remember me; but then, it was my breasts she was looking at, not my face.

Pushing Nicholas, I follow her down the familiar hallway to one of the examining rooms. "He'll be right with you," the receptionist says. Her eyes are full of professionalism, as Dr. S—'s employee.

Nicholas stirs in his stroller; seeing me, he reaches out his arms. I pick him up and put him on my lap. *I'm sorry,* I whisper into his soft cheek. *I should be taking you to a play class, or to the park.* I think, again, of leaving. This is my last chance, like on the ride at Disneyland. But if I go home to our quiet house, the silence will feel like deep water and what is there to keep me from drowning? I recall my mother's agonized lament before we moved to Hong Kong: "What will I do with myself?" Like her, I fear the places my mind wanders to when I'm idle.

"Hope!"

Dr. S— comes into the room, wearing his green surgical scrubs. In the harsh overhead light of the exam room, I see what it is about him that's different. Dr. S— has gained weight. At first, I think he's had a nose job, but I realize that his nose just looks smaller, in his rounded face.

He sits down on a stool with his hands beneath him, facing me. "So," he says. "You're married now, I take it."

"Yes."

"My wife is pregnant," he says. "With twins."

"That's wonderful," I say, even though he sounds tired, rather than excited, thinking about this.

"So what can I do for you today?"

"Um." My pants stick to my thighs as I rise off the table, putting Nicholas back in his stroller. "I want to ask you about my nose. There's a procedure you once recommended for me, in which a strip of cartilage is taken from behind the ear and inserted into the tip of the nose, to give it more, I think you called it 'projection'?" I change my statement into a question, because Dr. S— is looking at me incredulously.

"I would never recommend that for you," he says. "You're definitely not a candidate for that procedure."

"No? Really?"

Dr. S— leans forward, so that he is very close to my face. He reaches out and presses his finger to the skin between my nose and upper lip. "You have this *flatness* here," he says.

"Flatness?"

"Yes. Your upper lip has no roll to it." There is something dismissive in his tone. Could it be that I am less appealing to him now, slightly older, a wife and mother, no longer a fatuous young woman? He looks from me to my son. "Now *him*, on the other hand, he *would* be a candidate for that. You see that nice curve he has, just above the cupid's bow?"

I look from Dr. S— to my son's rosebud baby lips. I think, *No. It isn't possible. Not even Dr. S— would suggest plastic surgery for a six-month-old baby, would he? That can't be what he means.*

Dr. S—'s face is calm. Serious.

I want to laugh, suddenly, at the absurdity of this, of him. Of my being here. Dr. S— is looking at me, waiting for a response. It takes all my composure to say, "I see your point. Obviously, that procedure wouldn't work for me."

Dr. S— nods. "Well, it's nice to see you're showing good judgment now, not like before."

I stare at him, perplexed. Which of the procedures he performed on me did he consider "bad judgment"?

Dr. S— folds his arms over his chest, pushing back with his feet so that he shoots backward on his stool, kicking his legs out like a schoolboy. "Let's see those breasts," he says.

"I'm nursing," I say. "I've got pads in my bra. I can't take it off right now, I'll leak." Knowing he would ask me this, I have rehearsed what to say to him. I resolved, before coming here, that I would not take off my clothes for Dr. S—. It is one thing to be back in his office, without telling my husband where I am; it is another to disrobe for someone I once felt sexually attracted to, even if he is a doctor. It is a line I won't cross.

"I want you to know, Hope, that you're in a window of opportunity here. You could go bigger, if you want." Dr. S— holds his hands outstretched, to show the vast possibility. "My wife, Margo , is one who'll want to go bigger. It's very easy to do, at this point."

So he did operate on her, I think. *Poor Margo* .

"I have something I want to show you," he says. "Just wait here one second."

He darts out of the room, and I think, *I am not waiting here one more second. I'm leaving.*

I am maneuvering the stroller through the doorway, hoping to make a quick getaway, when Dr. S— appears again, out of breath, rushed. In one hand, he holds a large manila envelope, which he waves at me. A few papers stick out the top, as if he stuffed them in hurriedly.

"Are you late?" he says. Then, without waiting for my response: "Give me two seconds. You've got to see this."

I don't know if it's curiosity, or passivity, or just defeat that makes me come back into the room.

"This"—Dr. S— holds up the envelope triumphantly—"is a new procedure I've developed for the body. You could benefit from this. It's for women who've had children." He gives the folder an emphatic shake before handing it to me. "Take a look. I'm the only one doing this. You won't see this anywhere else!"

Reluctantly, I pull the papers out of the manila folder. Behind the typed pages are several large, glossy color photographs. I have to shake my head a few times to make sure I am seeing them right. The photographs are of the lower half of a woman's body, nude, on an operating table. Her pubic hair is matted with blood. Her legs are slightly splayed, in the inert posture of anesthesia. A few red smears stain the surgical paper between her thighs.

Oh, my God, I think. *Oh, my God.* Without looking at them again, I tuck the pictures under the papers and thrust them back at Dr. S—.

"So what do you think?" Dr. S— says jauntily, picking up the envelope and spilling its contents into his hands. "What I do is, I take fat from the buttocks and inject it into the labia. It increases sexual sensitivity and heightens orgasm." He speaks seriously, using his hands, as though explaining the procedure to a medical board. "It's revolutionary!" he says.

I want to say, *It's sick. You're sick.* But I can't. *Just pretend,* I think. *Like you used to. Act like you agree with him. Right or wrong, that is how you'll get out of here. Don't worry about being assertive now. Nod and smile and yes him.*

I can feel the spreading wetness beneath the arms of my blouse.

"Just *look* at this." Dr. S—, oblivious, presses some typed pages into my hands. A few words swim up at me, then dissolve: "increased sensitivity," "heightened sexual pleasure."

I feel a pressure building inside me, like a balloon inflating, pushing up my throat.

"I'm trying to get a patent," he says. "I've written to the *American Medical Journal.* The wonderful thing about this pro—"

"No!" I cry, so sharply that Dr. S— steps back a little. I thrust the papers back into his hands. "No. I'm not interested."

"Okay, all right." He shrugs, as if it is my loss that I do not want to hear about this. "You *will* want to think about it, though, after you've had more children. Everyone in town is going to want to do this."

He puts the papers and pictures in an untidy stack on top of the folder and puts the whole pile under his arm. "When you decide—"

There is a knock on the door. A husky, flirtatious woman's voice trills, "*Bob!*"

I move aside and Dr. S— opens the door to reveal a middle-aged woman in a tan jogging suit. She wears sunglasses and has a breathless, hurried air. "I just stopped in real quick," she says. "I was in the area. I thought I'd pop in and see what you have for me that's new and intriguing."

"Nina!" Dr. S— shows her his large, even teeth. "I'm so glad you're here. I've got some *great* new procedures I'm doing."

"Wonderful," breathes Nina.

I shudder, thinking of the photographs of the woman on the operating table.

"Hope here is just leaving," he says. "Why don't you come on in?"

As he holds the door for me to exit and Nina to enter, I notice one of the photos sticking out. I have a brief, terrible glimpse of pale skin, bloodied pubic hair, before Dr. S— closes the door.

I duck my head as I walk through the office area, striding briskly past the receptionist, who looks up expectantly. "Shall we set up your next appointment?" she asks.

At the door, I pause. "You don't remember me," I say. "But it doesn't matter, because you're never going to see me again." Her puzzled expression is the last thing I see.

In the backseat of my car in the dim underground parking lot, I nurse Nicholas. A kind of hysteria has overtaken me; I'm half crying, half laughing, shaking. I keep stroking Nicholas's hair, methodically, rhythmically.

I lean my head back and close my eyes. *Maybe,* I think, *there is a reason I came here today, after all. Maybe this is the closure I needed.*

Some minutes later, Nicholas is asleep, his mouth slipping away from my breast. Carefully, so as not to wake him, I put him into his car seat.

Turning out of the parking lot, the bright midday sun is a shock. Glancing in my rearview mirror, I see a hulking brown Rolls Royce behind me. I turn left out of the lot, the big car behind me. It's a kind of reflexive gesture, in Los Angeles, to see a fancy car and look inside to see if a celebrity is driving it. As I slow for a yellow light, the Rolls slides into the lane next to me. Through the tinted windows, I see that it is Dr. S—.

His head is turned away; his eyes skim appraisingly over a woman scurrying to cross the street, but apparently she does not measure up because he abruptly turns the corner in front of her. A blue handicapped plaque swings from his rearview mirror like a lolling tongue. How appropriate, I think. How utterly unsurprising. I picture him parking in a reserved spot at some restaurant or club, so that he won't have to walk, believing such privileges are his for the taking.

On Sunset Boulevard traffic lurches along slowly, caught in a lunch-hour snarl. Shimmery heat rises off the street in waves, turning the shiny cars into pieces of bright, hard candy. A black Range Rover inches up beside me. Glancing over, I am mesmerized by the beauty of the woman in the driver's seat. She has flawless porcelain skin, full lips, perfectly sculpted features. Her white-blonde hair is caught carelessly in a knot. She is the sort of beauty to which every superlative applies: stunning, ravishing, drop-dead gorgeous. A knock-out. Why is it, I wonder, that our descriptions of extreme beauty are synonymous with something cataclysmic, even fatal? I am able to stare at her openly because she is busy craning her neck to look at something. I follow her gaze to a billboard, high above the Sunset Strip. It is an advertisement for a late-night adult television program, featuring three barely dressed, voluptuous women with come-hither looks. It is impossible to tell whether it is a photograph or an artist's rendering. The women are so alike, except for the fact that one is a blonde, one a brunette, and one a redhead, they could either have been drawn by the same hand or sculpted by the same surgeon.

The woman beside me keeps staring, rapt, at the billboard. What is going through her mind? Is she jealous? Does she yearn to look like those women? Is she one of the women? It is impossible to say. She is so busy looking at the billboard that she does not notice the traffic surging forward. When the car behind her honks its disapproval, she startles.

I am suddenly, sharply aware of the irony of the moment, me

admiring her admiring them. To me, she is the ideal of beauty; if I looked like that, if my face were that perfect, there would be no room for improvement. I would be complete. Or would I? Do I really believe that anymore? *She* is staring at the women on the billboard, who might not even be real, and perhaps thinking the same thing. Isn't there always someone prettier, blonder, sexier, darker, younger, more appealing? A kind of ruthless food chain of perfection? I look around me: brilliant sunshine, shiny new cars, tanned and glorious people strolling the sidewalks. What ridiculous bounty. When anything is attainable, can we ever be satisfied? Is anything ever *enough,* in a culture built on the idea that either *I am perfect,* or *I am nothing*?

The traffic light changes, cars moving forward impatiently. Glancing again at the woman in the car beside mine, I think of how easily I can sink back into the quicksand of obsession. I can feel the old thought process roll into place; the anxiety of need quickens my pulse. It is, curiously, not mere envy which her beauty incites in me, but something more complex and insidious that makes her beauty both as alluring and as deadly as that of a Lorelei. Looking at her, I think: She is impossibly lovely, yes, but I am not *so* far from that ideal, am I? I *could* be that beautiful, with the right doctor, with the right amount of work, couldn't I?

I shake my head, hard, wanting to toss off the old, swampy pull of those thoughts. I turn onto Outpost and wind up and up and up into the Hollywood Hills. Finally I turn left on Mulholland, then right onto our street. At home, I lay Nicholas in his crib, propped with a rolled-up blanket on either side of his body the way the pediatrician recommended. Then I go into the kitchen, check the answering machine to see if anyone has called. My husband's voice is there, wondering where I am, asking whether I went to the Mommy-and-Me class I found out about, over at the YMCA in Burbank.

The empty feeling that overcame me this morning is still there, milder than before but still lingering. What is it telling me? What is underneath the surface chatter telling me to get my nose fixed, to find a plastic surgeon? I must listen more deeply than that.

I look around our house, at the pictures of the three of us, the furniture Ray and I have picked out together, the quiet evidence of a shared life. Am I quiet enough inside to listen now? What do I know for sure? Ray and Nicholas are everything to me; I wouldn't change the life I have now. But I need something more. More contact, more stimulation, more challenge. I need to see other people and get back into the flow of daily life. We can't exist forever in a humid cocoon of love, Nicholas and I. Just as he had to come out of me, so I, too, have to go out into the world. I need to get out the door, even if I'm fighting anxiety, and meet other mothers like myself. Perhaps I'll take a writing class . . . I can be a devoted wife and mother and still explore the things that matter to me, that make me whole, can't I?

But wait. There is something I must do first. I turn on the baby monitor and carry it out to the yard along with the phone. I want to lay down on the swing that hangs from the oak tree and feel the sun on my face while I call my husband. *I am here,* I will tell him. *I am home.*

CHAPTER 28

"Please check to make sure all the information on your wristband is correct," the woman at registration says.

I look down at the plastic hospital bracelet she is about to attach to my wrist.

"Date of birth is correct? Hope Donahue is spelled correctly?"

"That's me," I say, surprised at the brisk cheerfulness in my voice, which is completely at odds with how I feel.

"Your doctor is Arthur Scott?"

"Yes."

"You're here for a breast implant removal."

I nod. The woman wears a plastic name tag that says EVELYN. It droops to one side, and I imagine her pinning it on earlier that morning, in the dark predawn hours, hurrying to get ready for work.

"Someone will take you to a room so you can change for surgery," she says.

"Okay." I look across the room at my husband, who has folded himself into a chair by the door. His face is pale and drawn; there are dark circles under his eyes. Neither of us slept last night. Catching my eye, he smiles brightly and winks, giving me a thumbs-up sign. *He must really be nervous,* I think; I have never seen him give a thumbs-up sign to anyone.

This surgery is going to be both longer and more complicated than any I've had before. My breasts have become so encapsulated with scar tissue that the slightest touch causes me pain. I had to stop nursing Nicholas a month ago so that I would be dried up before the surgery. Even without milk in them, my breasts are hard and lumpy. When I run my fingers lightly over their surface, it feels like there are walnuts beneath the skin. This surgery is about more than just being in pain, though. This surgery is about reclaiming my body. I vehemently do not want these large, fake objects inside my body. To know this so definitely feels like a gift.

The doctor who will be removing them, Dr. Scott, is a referral from my OB/GYN. He devotes half of his practice to cosmetic work, the other to burn victims and children with congenital deformities. He is tall and kind, with a head of thick gray hair like a thatched roof. He told me that the surgery will take between four and six hours, during which I will be under general anesthesia. Dr. Scott has promised Ray that he will send a nurse out periodically to let him know how I am doing. Nicholas is at home with a trusted baby-sitter.

Evelyn shuffles papers on her desk while we wait for the orderly to arrive. Her flowered dress is rather low-cut; I can't help noticing that her own breasts are large and drooping and streaked with faint, purplish stretch marks like silt in a riverbed. Does it bother her, I wonder, that her body is less than perfect? Will it bother *me* when mine is, hours from now?

The orderly arrives, a surly-looking woman with dark hair pulled tightly into a bun. She stands beside my chair, waiting.

"Hi!" I say to her, sounding slightly hysterical. "How are you!" It occurs to me that I'm trying to be Miss Congeniality, as if by being very nice to everyone I can chock up some last-minute good karma and improve my chances of doing well during surgery.

Ray and I hold hands as we follow her down the long, off-white hall. "Is the surgery on this floor?" I ask, trying to make conversation.

"I don't know. I'd have to check with the nurse. Someone will tell you." She holds open the door of a small, white room, motioning me to enter.

"Thank you."

In the room's small bathroom, I take off my clothes and put on the white cotton gown, tying the strings behind my back. My hands are shaking. When I come out, Ray is sitting on the edge of the narrow bed, aiming a white console at the television on the wall, pushing the buttons violently. "Damn thing doesn't work," he mutters. I can see in his face how tense he is.

"I think it's this button," I say gently, adjusting his grip. "That one calls the nurse."

A morning talk show roars applause as a woman comes in to take my blood pressure. She seems kinder than the last one. "Do I have to take this off?" I ask, indicating the small gold locket around my neck, a gift from Ray. Inside are pictures of him and Nicholas.

She nods. "No metal. Sorry."

I undo the slender chain and hand it to my husband. He drops it into his shirt pocket.

"Wait," I say. "Let me have that back a minute."

I take the locket and press it to my lips.

The nurse squeezes my arm in a blood pressure cuff. It grips tightly, then releases with a long hiss. "Nervous?" she asks.

I nod.

Dr. Scott has told me that the reason the surgery will be so long is because he must be very careful to excise only the scar tissue, not the surrounding breast tissue. There are the usual risks associated with general anesthesia, as well as the risk of blood loss. Dr. Scott told me that I could, at the same time as this surgery, have my breasts lifted, even have a smaller implant put in, because without the implants I have now, my breasts are sure to be stretched out, flat, saggy. But I have declined either of these cosmetic options. I absolutely do not want more implants, even small ones, and having a breast lift increases the risk that I will not be able to nurse another child, something I hope very much to do. There is a chance, Dr. Scott says, that my postsurgical breasts may be slightly asymmetrical. Because of the size of my implants, he cannot tell just how much of my own breast tissue I have. "Those are awfully large implants," he said. "I'd say your breasts are at least seventy percent implant."

At least seventy percent, I think. What procedure was it that Dr. S— promised would improve my looks by at least seventy percent, a comment which made me feel only thirty percent attractive, only fractionally acceptable? Now, I would rather have sagging, asymmetrical, functional, real breasts than perfect, surgically enhanced fake ones.

"Why, if I may ask, did you decide to go with such large implants?" he asks.

"I really didn't decide on their size," I say. "I should have, but I didn't. I let the surgeon decide. Is it because the implants are so large that I've developed so much scarring?"

"Yes and no," he said. "All breast implants become encapsulated sooner or later, necessitating replacement. It could take ten or fifteen years, but sooner or later the patient will have to have them replaced. A responsible doctor will tell a patient this."

And a responsible patient would ask questions, I think.

"The fact that your implants were put in under the skin, instead of under the muscle, is also a factor," he said. "That's the easy way. The better, but more complicated, way to insert them is under the muscle. It depends on the doctor's skill level and how much effort he wants to make."

I showed Dr. Scott the scars in my hair, and told him about the short-lived "mini-lift."

"A mini-lift gives a mini-result. That's what I tell patients. What was the name of the doctor you went to?"

"Dr. S—," I said. "Bob S—." Dr. Scott shook his head, he didn't know him. Then something occurred to me. "He's not really a plastic surgeon. He's not board certified."

"Ah." Dr. Scott smiled wanly.

Now, another orderly arrives with a wheelchair to take me to the pre-op room. He is very old, with white hair and a distracted look.

"I don't need that," I say, indicating the wheelchair. "I'm fine to walk."

"Hospital policy," he grunts.

My husband and I exchange glances. Would it *kill* these people to be nice? Why is everyone here so brusque? Does living with life and death every day make you this careless and unflappable? I sit down in the wheelchair and try to rest my feet on the footrests, but they won't hold, flopping to the floor like trapdoors. The orderly reaches down and tries vainly to adjust them. Then he kicks at them with his foot, irritated. Finally they drop into place with a hollow metal thud. I put my feet on them, and he begins to push me down the hall. He walks surprisingly fast, considering his age and the burden of pushing me, and Ray has to hurry to keep up with him. I keep turning my head to make sure he is still there. I have given up trying to be nice to everyone. It doesn't matter anymore. My heart knocks hard in my chest, a trapped bird trying to beat its way out.

We arrive at two metal doors with a sign above them that reads SURGERY. The orderly presses a button and the doors swing open. He pushes me through briskly.

"You can't come in here," he says to Ray. "Patients only."

He doesn't stop pushing me as he speaks, so that I have to call over my shoulder, "Bye, Honey! I love you!" as Ray calls, "I love you too!" through the doors as they are closing. All I can see is a sliver of his white shirt and one raised arm, waving at me.

The pre-op room has five beds, with curtains that can be drawn around each one. I am in the second bed. None of the curtains are drawn, so I can see that all the other beds are empty except for the first one, where a man with a thick handlebar mustache snores softly. He has a green surgical cap on his head and an IV tube secured to his wrist with white tape. I wonder how long he has been there. It is so early in the morning.

The anesthesiologist comes in and introduces himself to me. He looks a little effeminate in his green paper cap, and this relaxes me, making me want to laugh. But when I see the bulge of a syringe in his pocket, the dread comes back.

He looks at my chart.

My mouth is dry. "So you've been doing this for years and years, right, and I have nothing to worry about?" I blurt.

"Years and years. Since eighty-two, if that makes you feel any better." He sounds tired, perhaps thinking about all those years.

"And I won't wake up in the middle of the surgery, right?"

"You won't wake up in the middle."

"Because I've heard that can happen, that you can wake up in the middle and not be able to move or speak or show you're awake, like a living nightmare." I'm babbling now, unable to stop myself.

"You've been reading something. Have you been reading something?"

"I heard about it on television, I think. A talk show."

"The only time that happens is when someone's been really injured, say in a car accident, and you can't give them too much anesthesia or they might die. But that won't happen to you."

"And you've done lots of cases like mine?"

"I'm vice chairman of the department."

"Oh. That makes me feel better." I am silent as he slides the thin IV needle into my arm, taping it in place. "So I guess there are a lot of people in here who are in worse shape than I am, huh?"

"I'd say there are a *lot* of people in here who are in a *lot* worse shape than you."

He's right, I think, chastened. I wonder if the man in the bed beside mine is one of them.

"I'll be back in a minute with something to help you relax," the anesthesiologist says.

I flip through the stack of magazines on the little stand by my bed. I can't concentrate. Panic grips me now, with its iron hand. I touch my breasts beneath the thin gown, feeling their hardness, the scar tissue that is threatening to pop the implants. *You did this to yourself,* I think.

The anesthesiologist returns with a syringe full of bright blue liquid.

"This will help you calm down," he says, injecting it into my IV tube, and as he speaks the drug enters my blood and my mind and my eyes become heavy.

"Ah. Yes," I say. The drug has taken effect so quickly that *yes* sounds like *yeth.* My tongue feels thick and seems to have swollen to fill my mouth. I am having trouble negotiating it in order to speak.

The anesthesiologist smiles, satisfied, then seems to go away. I hover in the neverland of half-sleep, too tired to lift a magazine off my lap. After a while, a blonde nurse appears and begins to fit my hair into a cap. Someone else is wheeling me into a brighter, colder room. The blonde nurse is putting blankets over my legs. She is talking to me as she works, the way a mother would talk to a frightened child, so soft and soothing that I want to cry. It's as if my own mother is thinking of me and speaking through this woman. *Honey, your hair won't even fit into this cap! You got some beautiful hair, you know that? Thick!* I smile, too tired to respond.

Sweetheart, you cold under those blankets? Let me get you some more. It is as if she appeared like an angel, to tell me all the comforting things I need to hear. Am I dreaming her? I try to focus my eyes on the woman's face but they keep falling shut. She has a soft Southern accent. *You sleep now, honey, just sleep. This will all be over before you know it. My sweet girl, you sweet thing.*

* * *

I awake in a white room on a narrow bed with my head propped up. My vision is blurry, but I am aware of lights overhead and noise and nurses walking around. I am shaking, the violent aftershocks of anesthesia. Someone comes and drapes a white blanket over my legs, which twitch and jerk like a marionette's. My teeth knock against each other.

I can tell from my restricted breathing that I am wearing a tight, corsetlike garment around my chest. Although my upper body is still numb, I have an odd but very distinct sense of having been handled, touched, and probed, as though my flesh has a memory and can recall what I do not. I lift my head to look around, and a wave of nausea overtakes me. I choke, vomiting into the blanket on my lap. There is nothing in me, only pale watery saliva, but I can't stop myself from gagging. I wonder vaguely if anyone notices. I can make out other beds in the room, other patients. I vomit again into the blanket, then try to wipe my face with it, but it is already soaked. I try to whimper, to signal someone's attention, but can't. I am underwater, unable to make a sound. Consciousness is something I can almost grasp, like reaching for a shimmery surface.

"Uh-oh, she's vomiting."

A nurse has noticed me and is coming closer. A plastic bin is handed to me and I vomit into it. Then I sink again, mercifully, into the dim underwater oblivion of sleep.

I awake again in a darker, quieter room. I have been moved to a slightly wider bed with metal arms on either side. A nurse is pouring water into a yellow pitcher. I see Ray sitting on a couch by a window.

"Honey?" he says, jumping up. "Hope? Are you awake?"

I try to sit up, but the pain in my chest is sharp as a dagger.

"How do you feel?" It is Dr. Scott, on the other side of me. He has the same kind expression he always wears, but there are dark circles under his eyes.

"I want to see them," I say. "Let me see my breasts."

"It's really not a good idea," he says.

"Please," I say. "Please, I just want to be sure they're there." I attempt a weak laugh, but the pain cuts me short, making me gasp.

Carefully, Dr. Scott undoes the tiny metal hooks along the front of the corset and holds it open for me, just enough so that I can look down.

My breasts are small and pale, sagging flat without the corset. A thin tube of clear rubber comes out the side of each breast, under my armpits. The tubes have plastic containers at the end into which a pinkish-red liquid drains. The horror of it fills me with terror, a terror that cuts through the drugs.

"I want to go home," I say. Suddenly, this is all that matters—getting out of the hospital. I look up at Dr. Scott, who is fastening up my corset, a crease of concentration between his brows. "You said I might be able to go home the same day. You said that."

"You really should stay overnight," he says. "It was such a long surgery."

"No!" I cry, each word a wince of pain. "I want to go home." A shudder of cold fear moves through my body. I feel like I might vomit again, and reach for the plastic pan by the bed. I retch into it, while my husband tries to hold back my hair. I am crying, my nose running down over my lips. "I want to go home," I sob, clutching the metal arms of the bed. "Please, Ray, please take me home."

My husband bites his lip. They are all looking at me, my husband, Dr. Scott, and a nurse, summoned by my vomiting; together, the three of them form a stern triptych around my bed. *Well,* I think. *If they won't help me, I'll get up myself.* I am aware of the absurdity of this: I am sweating and I have vomit in my hair and tubes coming out of my breasts but I am determined to go home. *I have to go home.* If I can leave the hospital, I can leave behind the pain and the fear and the horrible sight of my bound breasts. I try to sit up again, clutching the metal arms of the bed for support. With a yelp of pain, I sink back.

"You really need to stay here." The nurse speaks this time. I feel dizzy. They are talking to me underwater again.

"Why not stay?" Dr. Scott's voice now. "You can rest and you'll get your fluids and your antibiotics in the IV. You can have a sleeping pill and you'll wake up in the morning feeling much better. Why not stay?"

"Stay, Honey. Nicholas and I will pick you up at eight tomorrow morning."

From somewhere in my disorientation, my husband's words register. I blink, confused. "Is he . . . is Nicholas all right?"

"He's just fine," Ray says. "He misses his mommy, but he's fine. Your parents called, too."

A wave of fatigue washes over me. I am tired, too tired to speak. My eyes are falling shut.

"Just rest, Honey," Ray says. "We'll see you in the morning. First thing."

I am too tired to protest. I nod, then sleep.

I awake again sometime later to the sound of an agitated male voice somewhere nearby, in a room beside mine. A nurse stands beside my bed, taking my blood pressure. I have no idea what time it is. The light slanting through the window is the honeyed light of late afternoon. *Oh, God,* I think, my heart racing again with fear. *Oh, God, I've still got the whole night ahead of me.*

"Nooo!" the man next door is shouting. "No, don't touch me!"

"Who is that?" I ask the nurse, panicked.

"That's the man in three-fourteen," she says. "We're trying to get him settled. We were hoping he wouldn't wake you."

The nurse leaves, and I watch the last light reflected on the vast steel and glass building opposite my room, turning the colorless windows rosy and glimmering. I dread the fading light, dread it and welcome it both, because it means that time is, in fact, passing but also that the long, interminable night still lies ahead of me. The long night when I will likely lie unsleeping in this bed, alone, in pain and afraid.

I realize that the television is on. How did that happen? People chatter away pointlessly; a blurry laugh track gurgles in the background. Fumbling for the switch, I turn it off. The silence of the room is overwhelming. *Maybe I should call Ray to come pick me up,* I think. *No, he can't. He's home with Nicholas, it's too late to take him out. Besides, I'm supposed to stay here.* Fear settles in my body like treacle, making me feel heavy and stiff. I try to think of something to calm myself. I can think of nothing, I can't even conjure the image of my son's face. *Oh, please,* I think. *Please, God. Please help me.* I feel strange, sort of guilty, considering how infrequently I pray. But now, as the last light of day winks and twinkles on the building outside my window, I close my eyes and form in my mind and on my lips a silent request. *Just help me make it through this night.*

The door opens and another nurse comes in. This one has thick arms and two gold teeth. She is brisk and efficient and distant as she takes my temperature and asks if I have urinated. As she turns to leave, my heart lurches out after her.

"Wait!" What is her name? Nadine? Claudine? She turns expectantly. "Do I get more antibiotics in the IV?" I can't think of anything else to say. I don't want her to go, to leave me alone in this sterile, bare room.

"Nope," she says, glancing at my chart. "You can start them tomorrow, when you get home."

She turns to leave again and I want to reach out and grab her. "Wait!"

This time she looks annoyed.

"Um, do I have enough ice water?"

"You've got plenty. I'll check it again in the morning."

The morning! The door closes with a click and my heart seizes up with panic.

"Nooo!" the man beside me shouts. "*Nooooo!*"

My throat closes with fear.

I run my hands over the smooth, tight corset, beneath which my damaged body is beginning to heal. I breathe slowly, concentrating on the *in-out, in-out* of my breath.

And then, like a miracle, the strength and reassurance I prayed for is delivered. I can't explain it as anything other than a kind of divine gift. It is as if my fear peaks and then breaks, like a fever. I think, *My breasts may be small and flat now, but they are mine. My breasts, my body itself, is about so much more than just physical beauty. It has produced a child, nursed and nourished him. I am whole again now. I am myself.* Overcome with a feeling of calm, of peace, I buzz the nurse.

"I'd like my sleeping pill now, please," I say.

The pill is delivered, baby blue in its plastic cup. I swallow it with a sip of ice water and lie back on the pillow. Out the window I can see one of the giant billboards on Sunset Boulevard. It is an ad for Cirque du Soleil, surreal clown faces looming large.

Or is it the billboard with the three perfect, sexy women? As the pill takes effect, the colors seem to blur and shift so that I'm not sure whether what I see is beauty or parody, rouge and lipstick, or garish greasepaint. As I close my eyes, I realize this: It doesn't matter.

EPILOGUE

Maybe because I grew up in Los Angeles, I've always believed in Hollywood endings. I would like my own story to have such a finish, one in which everything is resolved and everyone goes off, permanently changed, into the sunset. I would like to say that I am no longer obsessed with my looks, that I never visited another plastic surgeon's office, that I never felt the compulsion to alter myself again. That would be a Hollywood ending. But it is not the ending of my story.

Here is the truth: I have changed. I can say with certainty that I will never again be in that small, dark, desperate place I was in twelve years ago. But do not think that I am completely "cured."

I have had, in no particular order, the following: collagen in my lips, twice; Botox in my forehead and around my eyes; permanent makeup tattooed onto my brows and my lips. Actually, I had my brows done once, decided I didn't like them, had the tattoos lasered off by a dermatologist, then redone by someone else. I even had a beauty mark tattooed by my eyebrow, and then I had *that* taken off. I have booked and then canceled four nose jobs. My obsession has been time-consuming and expensive. It has struck me as pointless and wasteful, and I have regretted these machinations I've put myself through. Botox froze my face into someone I did not recognize. My husband said that I lost my smile, because when you have Botox, your muscles are paralyzed and your eyes can't crinkle up and smile along with your mouth. There is also the unnerving fact, which I have never heard about or seen reported in all of the Botox articles, that when the doctor injects the botulism toxin, he or she uses a very thin needle which has to be pushed just a little bit into the bone, so that you hear a tiny shattering sound, like ice cracking. I am still, at times, bothered by what I see as the imperfections in my nose. I have had dozens of hair colors, cuts, and styles. My hair, my lips, and my beleaguered nose seem to be the features I concentrate most of my attention upon. My husband says that "my nose knows" when I am unhappy.

I have learned that my dissatisfaction with my appearance increases in direct proportion to how I feel. During times of grief or stress, I obsess. When I booked three of the four nose jobs I would cancel, I had recently suffered a miscarriage. Rather than deal with the pain inside me, I focused on my nose. I realized what I was doing, and went back to therapy for a while. The fourth time I booked a nose job, we had just moved from Los Angeles to New Jersey. My husband was still in L.A., tying up loose ends, and I and our four young children were living with my mother-in-law at her house for four months. On the surface, I did not show any signs of stress. People remarked at how smoothly I'd made the transition from West to East Coast. How was it, they wondered, that I could live in close quarters in someone else's house with so many small children and be so serene? Inside, though, I was not fine. My anxiety came back—it never fully goes away, but I can usually control it—and I began to focus on my nose again. Because I was exhausted all the time, I began to feel like a failure as a mother. I knew, even as I called for a consultation, that I was making a mistake. There is the expression about dragging your heels, but it was my heart I felt like I was dragging when I went to that office. I was halfhearted about what I was doing, almost brokenhearted. Inside, a voice was wailing that I shouldn't do this, I didn't *want* to do this. It was like I was marching myself to the gallows. But I went to see the doctor, I made the appointment for surgery, and then I backed out, all in quick succession. It was a useless exercise in distraction, and one I was deeply ashamed of. I particularly despise myself when my disorder takes me away from my children, whether mentally, physically, or emotionally. Every minute I spend either in a doctor's office or caught up in obsessing about my face is a minute when I could be interacting with them. When I'm obsessing, I am not present, neither to myself nor to others.

In 1997, after my second son was born, I suffered a severe postpartum anxiety disorder and my obstetrician placed me on a low dose of Prozac. My state of mind improved so dramatically that I decided to stay on the medication. Still, I did not, until about two years ago, think of my obsession as possibly something chemical. There were signs, though. I had begun writing short stories and sending them out to magazines. But before I sent out a story, I'd obsess over the first two or three sentences, changing and rearranging the words until my eyes crossed and I wept with frustration. It got to the point where I dreaded reading over my work, because I knew I would nit-pick every word. I remember thinking: *This is not normal. This is not just a writer's minute attention to detail.*

Then, after my daughter was born in 2001, I developed a new phobia: other people. I had always had some mild to moderate social anxiety, but now, whenever I had contact with another person, I would sweat profusely, feel faint and unreal. I dreaded picking my children up at school because I couldn't bear the thought of talking to the other mothers. I was angry and confused and paralyzed, and I had no idea why I felt that way. I would think to myself, *If only I could turn off my brain . . .* The same thing happened in the supermarket. Those few minutes in which I faced the check-out clerk were agony. I would have to change my blouse when I got home, because it would be soaked with sweat. It was too much. Something was not right, and I needed help. I had been in talk therapy off and on for years, but this, I sensed, demanded more.

It occurred to me one day that perhaps both my phobias and my obsessions could have something to do with an obsessive-compulsive disorder. I thought about how many "eccentric" relatives I had whose oddness might actually be pathology. On both sides of my family, people suffer from compulsions. My mother's father used to lock himself in the bathroom and mutter curses at himself. It was a family joke that if you walked past a closed door and heard "Pathetic chickenshit" or "Piss-ant loser," you knew who was in there. I see, now, that there really was nothing funny about this. It seems, almost, like a mild case of Tourette's. My father's mother rarely leaves the house. My father and his younger sister are hypochondriacs. My mother showers two or three times a day. The evidence was all around me, but I'd never put it all together before. And, like so many families, we fiercely resisted the label of mental illness. Perhaps, sometime in the near future, it will be no more shameful to say that one has OCD than it is to admit being a diabetic. For now, though, the stigma is still there.

It surprises me, now, that my therapist never observed this, although I know that she deliberately resisted putting a label on me that might contribute to my pathology, since I already had a tendency to think of myself as sick and damaged and incapable. But something told me, very strongly, that this might be a specific chemical imbalance. I got a referral to a psychiatrist and told him my story. I said, "I just want to get out of my own way and have a life. I want to stop being tangled up in my head, but I don't know how to stop. Do you think my condition has to do with OCD?" He said, without hesitation, "Absolutely." It was an enormous relief. I had always thought it was my fault—a weakness on my part—that I was so obsessed with my looks. Vanity. Conceit. Self-centeredness. These are all things I have been accused of. But the one truth about my condition which I didn't see for so long is the single most basic and astonishing: It was about much more than simply being beautiful. It was about having a compulsion to change myself and not being able to control my urge to do so. It makes sense to me, because even when I was beautiful—and there were times I knew that I was—the bad feelings didn't stop. I still felt anxious and self-conscious. Those feelings never went away, no matter how great I looked. In fact, they got worse, because I always imagined that people, other women in particular, hated me for being beautiful. My feelings about being beautiful and sexually appealing were so mixed up with guilt and shame, that alone had the makings of obsession. But that was only part of it.

The psychiatrist who diagnosed me with OCD put me on a much higher dose of Prozac. My phobias and anxiety and my obsessions with my looks lessened to the point where I functioned better than I ever had; I got so much more done because I was not borne down and exhausted by my thoughts all the time. But the anxiety and the obsession with my appearance has never gone away entirely. It did not magically disappear, *poof,* as I hoped it would, with either talk therapy or medication. It is my awareness of my disorder that has changed, not the disorder itself.

It is about more than just being beautiful. It seems so obvious now, but it took me twenty years to realize. Back when I gazed longingly at Brooke Shields's beautiful face, I equated beauty with safety, a security I did not feel at home or in the world. But feeling safe and whole has to come from within. It has very little to do with outer beauty. That fact is astonishing to me, but it is freeing, too. Profoundly freeing.

When I first started working on this book, someone asked me why I thought it was that I "chose" plastic surgery as my obsession instead of, say, anorexia or self-mutilation. Could it just as easily have been one of those, or was there something specific that propelled me toward plastic surgery? The answer is yes, there were specific factors. But they are not factors that apply only to me. It's become a cliché to blame the media, but the fact is that one does not have to grow up in Los Angeles to be bombarded with images and messages about perfect beauty and youth. The young, beautiful models in fashion magazines do not represent the norm. In fact, these freakishly beautiful women make up less than one percent of the population. Their looks are the result of a genetic gift. And yet, they are the standard against which we are told to measure ourselves. The magazines tell us that we, too, can be as lovely and desirable as they are if only we have the right beauty regimen, exercise program, or plastic surgery. And despite the bold claims of anti-aging treatments, there is no way to recapture youth. It's a profoundly unfair ideal that leads women on an impossible quest.

Even our most beautiful women feel inadequate. When Pamela Anderson had her breast implants taken out, I cheered along with so many others. Yet she subsequently had them replaced with even larger ones. In interviews, she claimed that she didn't feel like herself without big breasts.

The writer Olivia Goldsmith, who died recently while undergoing her eighteenth cosmetic procedure, wrote with wit and wisdom about the struggles women face. Her heroines lose their husbands to younger women and succumb to the pressures of Hollywood, even have endless plastic surgery, but in the end, they emerge triumphant and whole. They fight and win the very battles their creator herself struggled with. Sadly, Goldsmith's fictional creations arrive at a place of serenity which she herself ultimately could not.

Everyone's particular struggle is as unique as a fingerprint. It was not just societal pressure and a chemical imbalance that shaped my disorder. For me, as for everyone, there is the aspect of personal family history. My mother needed me to dazzle in a way she felt she did not. She both idolized and deeply resented my beauty. She wanted me to shine but she did not want to be outshone. As a young girl, I didn't know where my mother ended and I began— neither of us did—and I absorbed her aching, unmet needs for attention and approval. The simple recipe for my disorder, then, goes something like this: Take one part growing up in Los Angeles, add family history and upbringing. Add chemical imbalance and stir. Simmer over a period of years.

It's about more than just being beautiful. One look at Joan Rivers or Michael Jackson tells us that. But it's so easy to dismiss these people as parody, to say that they've become caricatures of themselves. We can say that they are simply crazy, or out of touch with reality, or guilty of extreme self-involvement. And they may or may not be all of those things. But when I look at Jackson's face, I shudder, not because he repulses me but because I understand what it is like to need to alter yourself so completely and relentlessly. I am willing to bet that he doesn't have any idea what he looks like when he sees himself in the mirror. I, too, once believed there was nothing about my physical self that was worth preserving. Given the chance to wipe off my features and start anew, I would have taken it. At a certain point, extreme self-scrutiny loses all perspective. I understand what it is like to focus solely on the outside of yourself, rather than the inside, which is not so easily changed. Being obsessive about anything, I think, is an outlet for misery. When I see Joan Rivers talking so openly about how she has her face touched up periodically, and how she has changed the shape of her eyes so that they look Asian, I see a person whose inner discomfort is so great that she can't keep her hands off of herself. People who bite their nails, pick compulsively at their skin, pull out their hair, starve themselves, have endless plastic surgery: It's all a matter of degree, a matter of choice and chance. If I had not been able to afford plastic surgery, would I have starved myself or traced a razor blade over my arm? I think so. I would have done *something* to myself. That I am sure of. Is plastic surgery the new self-mutilation? Perhaps.

It's about more than just being beautiful. It's about having all of these uncomfortable feelings inside you and not knowing how to express them or deal with them. Obsessions and other compulsive behaviors are about trying to control one's anxiety and/or depression by giving it a specific focus. And they work, at least for a time. Giving in to one's obsessive thoughts brings relief, albeit temporarily, the way a drink calms the drinker. Afterward, though, there are those feelings of shame, of embarrassment, of disgust with oneself. These feelings are particularly strong in me when I do something to myself which is less about changing my appearance and more purely neurotic. About a year ago, during a period of moderate but relentless stress, I shaved off my eyebrows. The idea to shave my brows had been rattling around in my mind for some time, and I knew it was sort of irrational, but I couldn't stop thinking about it. *What if I shaved off my eyebrows and re-drew them? How would I look?* Finally, in the shower one evening, I just gave in and did it. I looked freakish and felt ashamed. The same thing happened more recently. My husband was under a great deal of stress, we both were, and I impulsively shaved back my hairline about two inches. It looked ridiculous and I immediately regretted doing it. The only relief was that the compulsion to do it was gone. Again, it was an idea that had been circulating around in my head, my mind chanting, *Do it, do it.* It is particularly shameful and embarrassing to me to admit that I did these things, that I couldn't help myself. Anything that we do to improve our appearance, however extreme, is considered normal and acceptable. Doing something which damages your appearance, though, and not being able to explain why or to stop yourself from doing it, seems like the actions of a crazy person. It is far more *sick,* somehow, to admit to shaving off my brows and shaving back my hairline than to admit going to a plastic surgeon and asking for a slimmer nose. Consulting with a doctor seems sensible, rational. It was a very refined way to channel my obsession.

That's why, when I first told people about this book, I would say, *It's about my obsession with being beautiful.* It was easy to say, and easy for people to digest. *I was obsessed with my appearance.* What woman isn't? This confession always got a sympathetic response, particularly from women. *Oh yes, I had low self-esteem, I didn't think I was pretty enough.* Don't we all? What woman *doesn't* obsess over her appearance, at least sometimes? And it *is* about self-esteem, and the pressures society places on women, but for me to say that it's *only* about this, for me, is to take the easy way out, to ignore the darker truths of my disorder. Claiming that my obsession was only about being attractive is like saying that a diabetic's problem can be reduced to having a sweet tooth. It is about chemicals in the brain, specifically serotonin, and how they are being released and absorbed. We are at the mercy of these chemicals, like in a science-fiction movie where the giant robot's head pops open, revealing a little man at the controls. There is a form of OCD called body dysmorphic disorder, or "imagined ugliness," of which my condition has some elements. My obsession also resembles self-mutilation, as I said, and it bears similarities to trichotillomania, a disorder in which people pull their hair out, one strand at a time. This is a compulsion. It is not about low self-esteem. It has about as much to do with self-esteem as an egg has to do with a ham sandwich. Just as shaming and ridiculing (i.e., "guilting" a person into changing their behavior) doesn't work, so, conversely, all the talk therapy and esteem-building in the world will not stop that voice telling you to draw your own blood or to pluck out your hair. That's the little guy in the brain. For as long as those neurotransmitters are malfunctioning, the compulsion, whatever it is, will be there.

I watch my children for signs of OCD. I have a son who is very concerned with germs and I keep an eye on that, while being careful not to shame him or make him self-conscious about it. As for my daughter, who is only two, I will watch her perhaps most closely for signs of distress, particularly regarding her appearance. Having a daughter of my own makes me realize how deeply my parents must have been hurt when I underwent plastic surgery. Every parent sees her child as beautiful and perfect, and it would be a knife in the chest for any of my children to want to cut into themselves. I am afraid of even piercing my daughter's ears for fear that she will begin to get the message that she needs to change herself to be beautiful. I am very glad that we live far from Los Angeles.

I would be wary of ever calling myself "cured" of my disorder because I'm afraid to perch myself atop that smug, lofty wall. It is better for me to be reminded of my own frailty; it gives me compassion not just for myself but for others, for anyone who is in pain.

I used to be terrified of my own weakness; if I acknowledged it, I thought I would be overwhelmed by it. But I am stronger and braver than that. I am not so easily broken. I am strong enough to realize that it is all right to be fragile, to be less than perfect. Staying connected to that vulnerability, ironically, gives me strength.